Chemical Communication

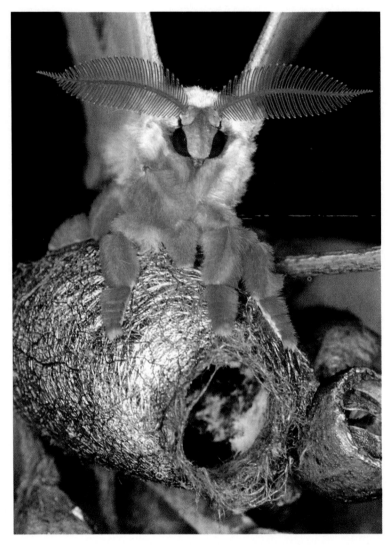

A newly hatched male gum emperor moth. The male senses
the presence of a female by detecting her pheromone with his
large, feathery antennae.

CHEMICAL COMMUNICATION

The Language of Pheromones

William C. Agosta

SCIENTIFIC AMERICAN LIBRARY

A division of HPHLP
New York

Library of Congress Cataloging-in-Publication Data

Agosta, William C.
    Chemical communication: the language of pheromones / William C.
Agosta.
        p.   cm.
    Includes bibliographical references and index.
    ISBN 0-7167-5036-8
    1. Pheromones.   I. Title.
QP572.P47A4   1992
591.59—dc20   92-9412
                                                                           CIP

ISSN 140-3213-5026-0

Printed in the United States of America

Scientific American Library
A Division of HPHLP
New York

Distributed by W. H. Freeman and Company
41 Madison Avenue, New York, NY 10010
20 Beaumont Street, Oxford OX1 2NQ, England

2 3 4 5 6 7 8 9 0   KP   9 9 8 7 6 5 4 3 2

This book is number 41 of a series.

CONTENTS

PREFACE

$\mathcal{A}$bout twenty years ago, some of my colleagues in another laboratory at The Rockefeller University were investigating the Syrian golden hamster. They were using the hamster's sex attractant to explore biological and behavioral questions, and they recognized that knowledge of the chemical compounds responsible for the hamster attractant could facilitate their research. No one had ever examined this pheromone chemically, and they soon found that doing so would require a serious chemical investigation. At this point they encouraged my research group to take up the problem.

Now, my research group spent all its time exploring details of how chemical reactions work. Although we were very familiar with handling chemical compounds, we had never dealt with chemical signals or hamsters. Working with chemical reactions seemed quite different to me from investigating small rodents. Nonetheless, the idea intrigued me, because at that time no one knew much about the chemistry of mammalian pheromones. I was interested and agreed to plunge in.

In making this decision, I understood that our investigation would move much faster if the experiments were in the hands of someone already experienced with pheromones. I began looking for an investigator with an appropriate background and very soon found just the right person. Dr. Alan G. Singer had just completed his doctoral research, isolating and identifying a mammalian pheromone, and the experience had given him ideal preparation for the hamster problem. I persuaded him to join us at Rockefeller as a postdoctoral fellow and to devote his full attention to the hamster attractant. Over the next two years he first determined the identity of the major hamster sex attractant and then turned his attention, with similar success, to another signal that is a powerful aphrodisiac for the male hamster.

Our accomplishments rightly reflect Singer's ability and effort, but they also owe a great debt to an unusually effective interdisciplinary collaboration with two groups of biologists. Because no one is equipped to work equally well in all the areas that contribute to the study of pheromones, cooperative research has had an important role in understanding chemical communication.

The scientific study of pheromones combines elements of several disciplines, but many of the results can be understood and discussed without much technical language. This volume brings together information about chemical signals that carry a wide variety of messages in species from microbes to man. No particular knowledge of animal behavior, sensory physiology, or organic chemistry is required to follow the discussion, although enough technical detail and reference material are provided to permit the prepared reader to explore further. I have presented the chemical structures of the compounds responsible for many of the pheromones discussed, even though we do not yet understand much about why one structure and not another serves to carry a specific chemical message. I appreciate that most people (including scientists in many other fields) do not share the organic chemist's strong esthetic sense for molecular structures, but for me the story of pheromones would have been incomplete without their chemical identities. Of course I hope that you will agree, but a reader less enthusiastic about chemistry should be assured that many behavioral scientists pursue significant research into chemical communication without giving more than a passing thought to chemical structure.

Discussions of pheromones can be organized around either messages or organisms. I suspect that for most people biological species are more familiar than the signals these species use, and for this reason I have organized the discussion around organisms. This approach also emphasizes the grand sweep of diverse living creatures that make use of chemical communication. I have started with more simply organized species and moved toward more complex ones. Some scientific problems associated with chemical signals grow more difficult as the organisms using the signals become more complex, and moving toward increasing complexity provides a gradual approach to these difficulties.

I began writing this book wondering whether it would find an audience. The subject attracted me, but had enough people heard of pheromones to be interested in reading about them? I was recently reassured on this point. When two New York socialites kissed and made up immediately after a well publicized spat, a local gossip columnist explained confidently that it was "a chemical thing involving pheromones." This disclosure came to my attention, and I was delighted to learn that chemical signals had achieved such a prominent place in the world. This should certainly be an appropriate time to say something serious about them.

William C. Agosta
New York, March 1992

Chemical Communication

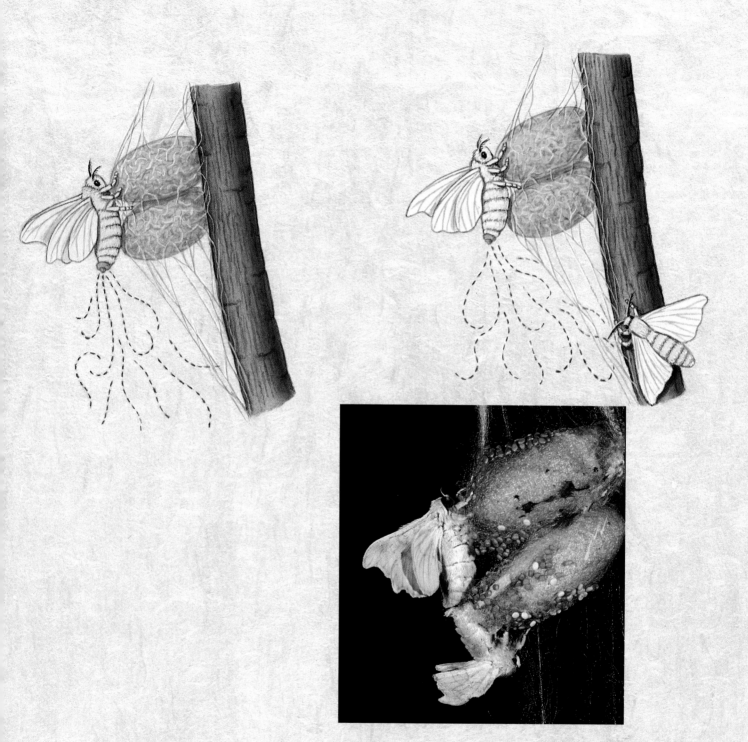

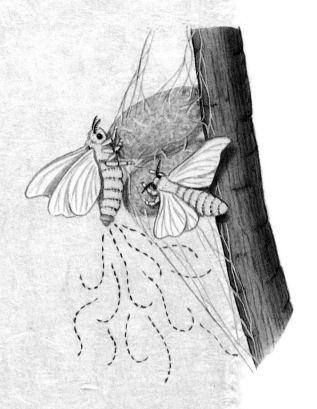

■ A female silkworm moth, perched on a cocoon, emits a chemical signal that attracts a mate. So small is the amount of chemical produced that to isolate and identify the substance scientists needed twenty years and over half a million female moths.

1

MOLECULAR MESSENGERS

*H*uman beings gather information about the outside world largely through sight and sound. These are our best-developed senses, and when we want to know what is going on we look and listen. For many other living creatures, the world is a much different place: for them chemical signals are the primary source of information. Chemical compounds from other organisms or events in the environment provide their basic knowledge of the world. Even many creatures that do have other well-developed senses find chemical signals to be indispensable. Species as diverse as water molds and elephants depend on the ability to sense chemicals in the world around them for survival. Even simple bacteria respond efficiently to certain chemicals, moving toward foodstuffs and away from toxic compounds. Humans must have developed an early appreciation of chemical signals. The attraction of a male dog

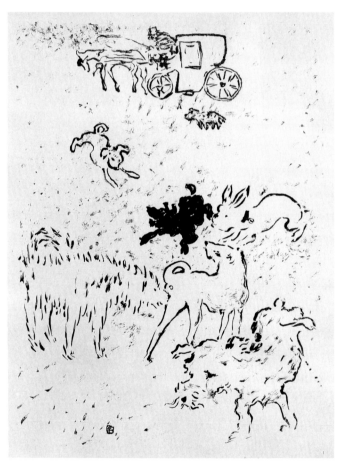

Dogs commonly sniff at one another, as depicted in this lithograph by Pierre Bonnard. They are a thousand to a million times more sensitive to various odors than we are, and recognize each other by smell.

to a female, for example, could have provided important clues thousands of years ago. Even earlier, hunters must have learned about the significance of scent to both prey and predator. However, our organized, scientific understanding of chemical signals is a much more recent development. This understanding began in the nineteenth century with the experiments of naturalists who were intrigued by the ability of female moths and butterflies to attract the male. For decades these investigators documented attraction for various species, often over distances of several kilometers. Through clever experiments they demonstrated that functional antennae were critical for the male to locate the female: males could no longer find females when their antennae were covered with lacquer or totally removed.

These observations were fascinating, but scientists achieved a satisfactory interpretation of them only slowly. Initial explanations invoked some sort of radiation from the female, and one idea was that the male's antennae were appropriately tuned to receive the wavelength broadcast by the females of his species. As late as 1950, investigators found that infrared radiation emanated from the region of the thorax of females of two species of moth. In their report of this discovery, these scientists wondered if this radiation might be the signal emitted by the female to lure her mate.

On a more rewarding track, as early as the 1930s there were reports of the extraction of "attractivity" from female moths. There was also evidence that attractive substances were present in the air over cages containing females. Experiments eventually showed convincingly that attractivity must be due to volatile chemical substances. At the end of the 1930s this conclusion was firmly enough established that the German chemist and Nobel laureate Adolph Butenandt became interested in undertaking the isolation and identification

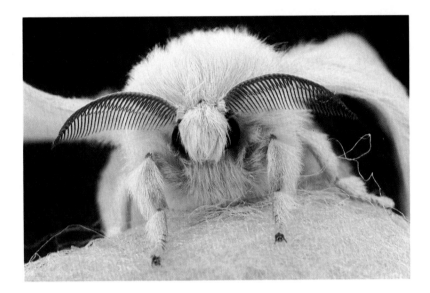

About half the 15,000 to 20,000 hairs on the feathery antennae of a male silkworm moth are specialized for detection of the sex attractant released by the female.

of such a sex attractant. After some twenty years this research led to the identification of bombykol, the sex attractant of the female silkworm moth *Bombyx mori*. This investigation holds an important place in our understanding of pheromones, and we shall return to it later.

At about the time that Butenandt completed the work on bombykol, Peter Karlson and Martin Lüscher coined the word *pheromone* to describe a chemical signal transmitted between members of the same species. (The word was created from two Greek words, *pherein*, to transfer, and *hormon*, to excite.) They wished to distinguish pheromones from other kinds of chemical signals that convey information to organisms. Some of these other kinds of signals come from whole systems such as rivers or forests, as when the odor of its native stream guides a salmon returning after years in the distant ocean. Other chemical signals pass from members of one species to another: dying trees release substances detected by bark beetles that then attack the trees;

skunks defend themselves against other animals with an unforgettably malodorous spray. None of these examples concerns a message sent and received within a single species, and so none of these signals is a pheromone. There is also another kind of chemical signal that is not a pheromone, even though it does concern a single species. This is a signal that operates within a single individual, delivering a message from one part of the organism to another. These signals are known as *hormones*, and they will turn up again later in our explorations.

While Butenandt was setting out to isolate bombykol, the famous behaviorist Karl von Frisch was making one of the classic discoveries of chemical communication. An Austrian zoologist most widely known for his work with honey bees, von Frisch (1886–1982) shared in the Nobel Prize for Physiology or Medicine in 1973. His contribution to the study of pheromones emerged from his work with the European minnow *Phoxinus phoxinus*, and it came about through two casual observations. The

A school of young European minnows.

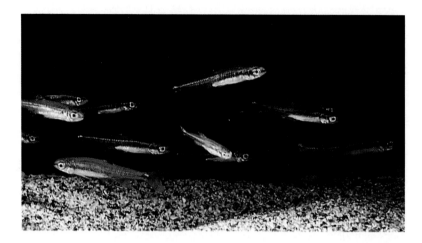

first concerned a minnow that von Frisch had marked with an incision near its tail. When he returned this individual to the school, the other minnows became frightened and some of them retreated. The second observation followed von Frisch's finding a minnow stuck under the rim of a feeding tube, struggling to free itself. He released the fish, and when it swam away toward the group, they all fled in fright. To von Frisch these episodes were curious enough to warrant detailed investigation, and his carefully documented results set the direction of much later research into chemical communication in fishes.

Von Frisch called the agent responsible for this fright reaction the "alarm substance." Subsequent work has shown that most members of this group of fishes (the ostariophysians) show a fright reaction when an injured ostariophysian is introduced into the water nearby; the nature of the reaction itself varies with species, sex, and location of the reacting fishes. They may swim in a tighter school, leap at the surface, swim away and hide, or sink to the bottom and become very still. In some instances they will avoid the area of their disturbing encounter for some time thereafter. In at least one species the fright reaction changes over the life of the fish: young creek chub (*Semotilus atromaculatus*) dart away and hide, but adults drop quietly to the bottom and remain motionless.

This sudden and remarkable reaction is under the control of a pheromone in the skin of the fish, where it is carried in large alarm-system cells. These cells are fragile, and upon injury they rupture, discharging the pheromone into the water. Simply scaring a fish does not affect its alarm-system cells, but even minor mechanical damage to the skin will disrupt them, and damage to only a small area of the skin of a single fish is capable of causing fright in an entire school.

The alarm substance and bombykol are just two of thousands of pheromones. All sorts of organisms use chemical signals to convey a rich variety of messages. The alarm substance signals "danger—get out of here!," and bombykol is the female moth's message "come to me." Other pheromones bear messages such as "the queen is in the hive and all is well," "produce more sex hormone," "we are under attack!" and "I am pregnant." Messages may elicit a specific behavioral response in the recipient, such as swimming toward the source of the signal or attacking an enemy. Alterna-

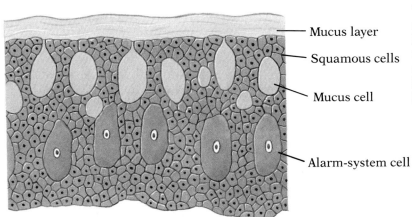

The large alarm-system cells of the European minnow are located in the outer layer of the skin, where they can be ruptured easily upon injury. The mucus cells discharge the slimy substance that forms the protective outer coating of fish.

tively, the message may cause a physiological change in the recipient, perhaps altering the timing of the sexual cycle or inducing puberty. For some species we are aware of only one pheromone and a single message. Other species, such as ants and honey bees, use many different chemical signals to coordinate the activities of their complex communities.

As we consider the significance of pheromones in the living world, it is important to keep in mind that human beings make relatively minor use of the ability to sense chemicals in the environment. Our primary means of detecting chemicals is through olfaction, the sense of smell. The sensitive discrimination of professional perfumers and wine tasters demonstrates that considerable refinement of the human olfactory ability is possible, but we are much less sensitive to chemicals than many other species. It is quite normal for some people to be a thousand-fold more sensitive than others to specific chemicals, evidence of how variable the importance of olfaction is to humans. Without a sense of smell, we would certainly find the world a much poorer place, but for us olfaction is not critical to survival or even to a reasonable existence. People who lack a sense of smell are said to suffer from

anosmia. This condition accompanies several serious maladies, but there are many anosmic people who show no other defect and who live quite normal lives. For human beings, anosmia is not even remotely comparable to the losses entailed in blindness or deafness. In contrast,

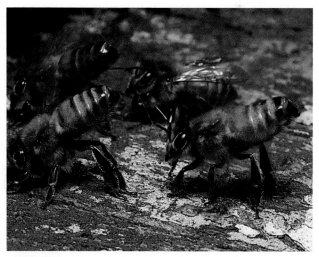

When disturbed, honey bees release an alarm pheromone and fan their wings to disperse the signal to their nest mates.

chemical communication plays an indispensable role in the lives of the creatures that we shall discuss in the pages that follow.

Pheromones as Chemical Compounds

Pheromones are specific chemical compounds or mixtures of compounds. This means that they are real objects that are endowed with definite physical and chemical properties. Once released, a pheromone has a physical existence quite apart from the organism that produced it. A volatile chemical signal may be carried on the breeze or in a current of water, to deliver its message at a later time and in a place remote from its source. Such a signal could be effective at attracting faraway mates or helpers. Chemical signals may also be persistent. Some of them can be deposited on a bush or on the ground, to be detected where they were left after the sender has departed. If such a signal is chemically stable and not too volatile, it may remain in place, and active for days. Stability and nonvolatility are good properties for a signal used, for example, to delineate the boundaries of a territory or to mark a food source. Conversely, the signal may be chemically unstable and destined to provide its message only briefly. This might be useful in a pheromone employed to give an immediate and short-term warning of danger.

Pheromones that travel through the air need to be volatile, ones that are released in the ocean must be stable in water, and ones that must remain in one place for an extended period should be persistent. Virtually all the compounds that will appear in the pages to follow are organic molecules. Molecules are groups of atoms assembled into a specific three-dimensional arrangement or structure, and *organic* simply means that these molecules contain carbon atoms. Properties such as volatility, persistence, and stability have their basis in molecular structure. The smaller a molecule of a given kind of is, the more volatile the compound will be. Two simple molecules illustrate the effect of size: pentane has 5 carbon atoms and pentadecane has 15, but

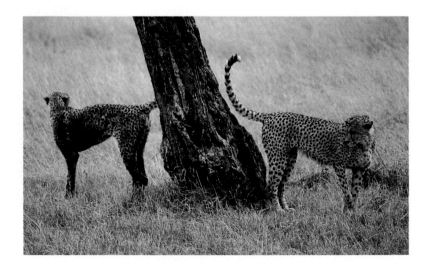

Like many other cats, cheetahs (*Acinonyx jubatus*) send a spurt of urine backward to mark trees and other conspicuous objects. This probably permits small groups of cheetahs to avoid each other while hunting in the same range.

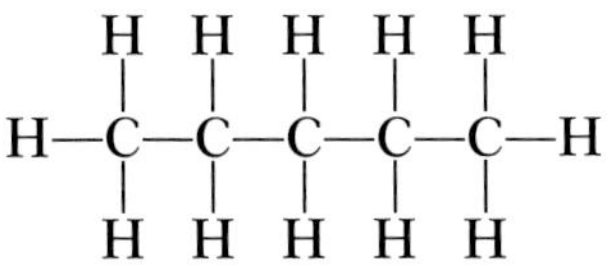

Pentane

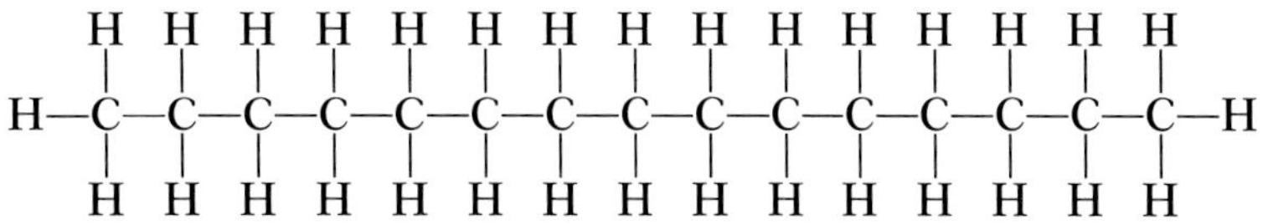

Pentadecane

In discussing the structures of molecules, it is convenient to write down structural formulas, using a symbol for each atom and showing specifically how the atoms of the molecule are interconnected. The symbols for the atoms we generally need are just the first letter of the name of the element: H for hydrogen, C for carbon, O for oxygen, N for nitrogen, and S for sulfur, for example. Each line connecting the symbols represents a bond joining two atoms.

otherwise they look much alike; yet the small size of the pentane molecule leads to high volatility. A small amount of pentane poured into a saucer will evaporate in a minute or so, whereas the much larger pentadecane molecules form an oily, persistent substance. A small amount does not evaporate noticeably in hours.

Volatility and persistence also reflect the *functional groups* present in a molecule. These are groupings of atoms that appear repeatedly in the structural formulas of organic compounds; they are attached to or embedded in a framework of carbon atoms. Several of the most common ones are illustrated below:

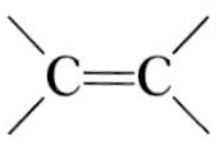

Carbon-carbon double bond

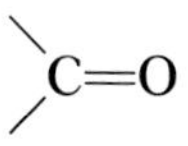

Carbonyl group

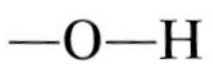

Hydroxyl group

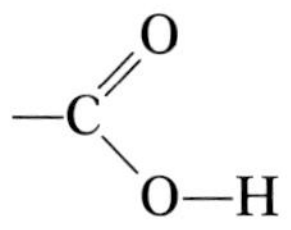

Carboxyl group

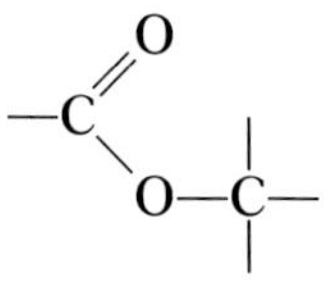

Ester group

The double lines indicate that atoms are connected by two bonds, called a double bond. Because double bonds are flat and rigid, functional groups help determine the shape of molecules. Groups of atoms can twist about single bonds, but the two atoms bonded by a double bond remain rigidly bound.

This property of double bonds has an interesting consequence. There are two possible arrangements of two atoms attached to opposite ends of a carbon-carbon double bond, called *E* (from the German *entgegen*, opposite) and *Z* (from the German *zusammen*, together). Older names for these two arrangements are *trans* and *cis*, respectively. The two forms of 2-butene are two different chemical compounds, and each has characteristic chemical and physical properties.

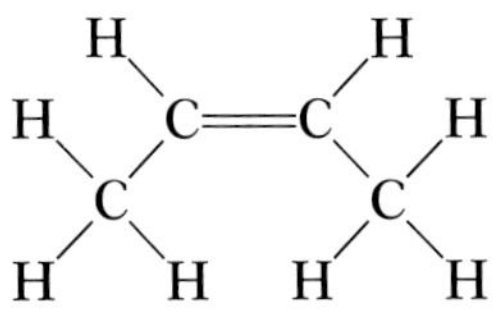

Z-2-Butene

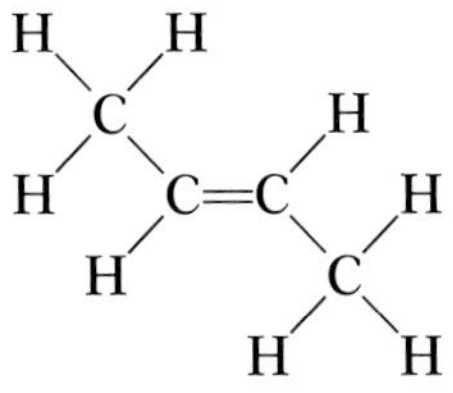

E-2-Butene

The effect of functional groups on volatility is well illustrated by the two compounds propane and propanol. These two compounds differ by only one oxygen atom, but this atom is part of a hydroxyl group, and its presence has a striking effect on volatility. Propane is much more volatile than pentane, but propanol is much less so. The hydroxyl groups in different molecules of propanol interact with one another and reduce its volatility. Propanol behaves like a larger molecule than it is.

Functional groups are sites of reactivity in a molecule. They make new bonds with various other molecules and ions (atoms or groups of atoms that carry electrical charge), and the strength of their tendency to form bonds determines whether a compound is reactive or inert, stable or unstable. These are relative terms: a molecule with functional groups that react with water but not with dry air would be unstable in the ocean but could be stable in the desert. The alarm pheromone of a minnow has functional groups that make it reasonably stable in water, whereas the attractant of the golden hamster has functional groups that

$$H_3C-CH_2-CH_3$$

Propane

$$H_3C-CH_2-CH_2-OH$$

Propanol

The formulas for propane and propanol, and other compounds, can be written in a more compact way by eliminating the bonds between C and H.

make it reasonably stable in the hamster's desert home.

Throughout the natural world a wide variety of molecules serve as pheromones. Totally different kinds of molecules bear qualitatively similar messages in different organisms, and there are no obvious rules about the structures used. Beyond commonsense requirements that a pheromone be suited to its environment, there is no simple way of predicting the sort of molecule a particular species may use for carrying a message. The only way to find out what compounds are acting as pheromones is to isolate and identify them chemically. This was Butenandt's goal in working with bombykol, and it remains the main chemical problem in pheromone research today.

The Scientific Study of Pheromones

In the years immediately after the success with bombykol, the study of pheromones achieved wide popularity. Our present knowledge in this area results from thousands of separate studies over the past thirty years. Pheromones are extremely widespread in nature, and scientists have studied the pheromones of animals, algae, fungi, and bacteria. Very little is known about whether plants use chemical signals, although there is one tantalizing report that points to pheromones in poplar and maple trees. Most of the current fund of knowledge comes from work on insects, followed distantly by work on mammals.

Studies of pheromones usually begin with a simple observation. That is, when presented with the putative signal, the organism under study changes physiologically or behaviorally. There are many reports that have not yet been carried further than this. Dealing with such observations over the years has instilled caution in interpreting them, and usually the next step is to design and carry out more extensive experiments with careful controls. In favorable circumstances these experiments establish a clear connection between a signal from one organism and its reproducible effect in other members of the same species. Much of our present knowledge is at this level. Once the existence of a pheromone and its effect is firmly established, investigations may go in various directions, from group behavior to neurophysiology to genetics, with the aim of understanding the pheromone more fully from various points of view and of fitting it into a larger body of behavioral and biological knowledge. At this point there may also be an effort to identify the chemical compounds responsible for the pheromonal effect.

Identifying these compounds requires separating them from the natural mixture or secretion in which they occur. The systematic separation of a mixture of chemical compounds into its pure components is called fractionation. Chemists take advantage of differences in the chemical and physical properties of the components of a mixture to partition these components between two or more states. This partitioning may be between liquid and vapor, or solution and solid, or solution and adsorbent, among other possibilities.

A chemist who wishes to identify the active compound or compounds in a pheromone often begins with the total contents of a gland that makes and stores the pheromone, or perhaps he begins with gallons of seawater containing the pheromone along with hundreds of other components. He must have available a wide assortment of procedures for fractionation, because pheromones include compounds with many different sorts of chemical and physical properties. The chemist may require many steps and several different procedures to purify the compound or compounds responsible for the chemical signal.

Fractionation techniques can be effective only if the investigator has some means of following his progress. After performing a separation step, he must answer such questions as: Did the procedure work? In which fraction or fractions is the desired material? How much purer is the desired material now than before? An assay is essential, and ideally it should be quick, cheap, and dependent in a known fashion on some property of the compound being isolated. If the compound is a pheromone, the only property initially known to the investigator usually is its biological effect on the natural recipient. The investigator needs some sort of procedure that uses this biological effect to guide his fractionation, and this procedure is a bioassay. An obvious way to follow the isolation of a sex attractant, for example, is to gauge the attractivity of fractions by testing them on the natural recipient of the pheromone. To evaluate a sample's attractivity, the investigator will normally score or time some activity, such as movement toward the sample or the beating of an insect's wings.

Once the investigator has the pure components in hand, he can identify them. For each component, he must establish the number and position of the atoms present in its molecules. Structure determination, as this is called, relies on a combination of chemical and physical techniques. By carrying out chemical reactions and physical measurements on the compound, the chemist can obtain a complete count of all atoms present, determine the carbon framework of chains and rings, and identify and locate all functional groups.

Nearly always, the chemist working with pheromones must isolate, purify, and identify

CHAPTER 1

An original sample containing a pheromone is separated into different fractions according to some chemical or physical property. Each fraction is tested in a bioassay to determine which one (or ones) carry the pheromone. If the pheromone is concentrated in a single fraction, this active fraction is then separated once again according to some other property, and the bioassay is repeated. Obtaining a pure pheromone may require many cycles of fractionation. The fractions that do not carry the pheromone can be discarded.

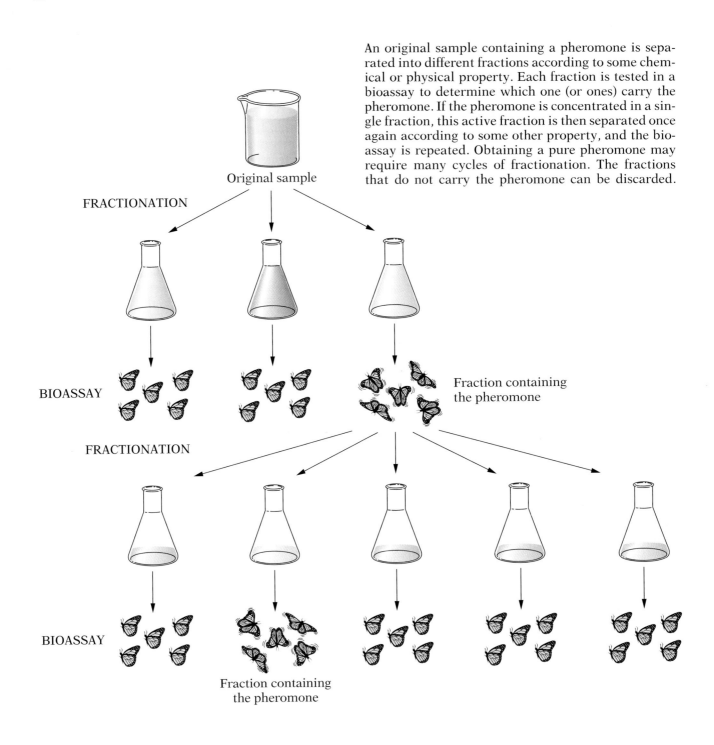

Original sample

FRACTIONATION

BIOASSAY

Fraction containing
the pheromone

FRACTIONATION

BIOASSAY

Fraction containing
the pheromone

compounds that are available only in minute amounts. One of the most frequent observations in this area is that all kinds of organisms are exquisitely sensitive to their pheromones. Often only a minute amount of material is necessary to send a chemical message, even to a large number of recipients. Consequently, an organism may never keep more than a little of the pheromone on hand. A female silkworm moth ordinarily contains enough bombykol to excite many millions of males, but this requires only about 1.2 micrograms of material. Moreover, even the most skilled investigator loses material during isolation and purification, and so only very small amounts of most pheromones can be obtained for chemical study. In early years this was a technical barrier that virtually prohibited rigorous chemical identification of pheromones. Butenandt and his group had about 6 milligrams of bombykol available for its identification in the 1950s, and they were forced to devise novel methods to solve the problem. Fortunately, owing to technical improvements over the years, scientists can purify and identify ever smaller amounts of material. A present-day chemist could probably identify bombykol using less that a hundredth as much material as Butenandt needed. Some substances can now be identified from samples of only a few picograms.

With a knowledge of the chemical constitution of a pheromone, new research problems present themselves. How does the organism transform chemical compounds in its diet into the pheromone? How does the pheromone deliver its message to the recipient? Answers to such questions depend on knowing what the pheromone is, that is, on knowing the chemical structures of its components. At present, structures are available for only a small fraction of the pheromones that have been described.

An Interdisciplinary Effort

The study of pheromones is an area of scientific research that draws information, techniques, and investigators from behavior, biology, and chemistry. One of the attractions here is the opportunity to work collaboratively with scientists who are trained in other disciplines and who sometimes bring a quite different perspective to a shared research problem. Few investigators are equipped to work equally well in all these areas, and interdisciplinary cooperation can be especially fruitful.

In the pages that follow we shall sample what is known about pheromones in water molds, insects, mammals, and many other creatures, drawing largely on examples where behavior, biology, and chemistry have all contributed to our current knowledge. We cannot discuss all that is known, but we will explore many kinds of organisms and their chemical signals and also have a look at how scientists go about their research in this area. We start with simple organisms and then move through the animal kingdom to the mammals. In the final chapter we consider the provocative question of pheromones in humans.

It is certainly possible to appreciate the fascination of pheromones without a detailed knowledge of the disciplines that contribute to their understanding. A number of terms, concepts, and techniques come up repeatedly, and the glossary following Chapter 7 contains definitions and brief discussions that may clarify these matters.

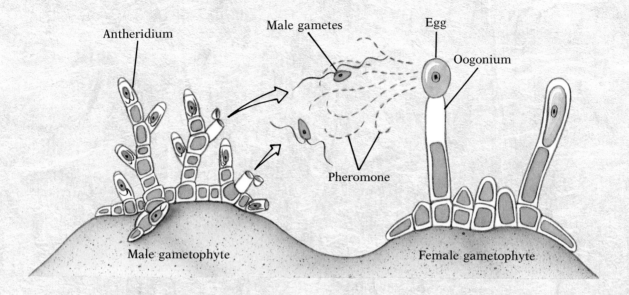

Antheridium

Male gametes

Egg

Oogonium

Pheromone

Male gametophyte

Female gametophyte

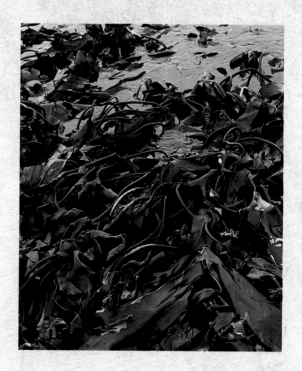

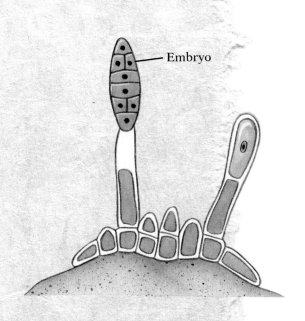

Embryo

■ A pheromone ensures the union of sperm and egg in the brown alga *Laminaria digitata*. The large masses of this seaweed seen along North Atlantic coasts are the asexual form of the alga. Its spores give rise to microscopic sexual forms, called gametophytes. The gametes (eggs) of the female gametophyte release a pheromone that attracts male gametes (sperm). The embryo produced by their union will eventually grow into the thick blades and stalks of the asexual form.

2

NAVIGATING BY PHEROMONES

From a chemical point of view there is no such thing as a simple biological system, but certain molds, algae, water molds, and bacteria do offer simplifications that make the study of their chemical communication relatively straightforward. In some of these creatures, the sender and receiver of the pheromonal message are just two cells rather than entire organisms. The species that we will discuss live in water, and some of them eject male and female reproductive cells, or gametes, that must find each other in the water for fertilization to take place. To improve their chances of fertilization, one of the gametes releases a pheromone that attracts gametes of the opposite sex. Unlike the situation in complex multicellular organisms, the response of a single gamete need not be coordinated with the activities of other cells and tissues or adjusted to benefit a large cellular community.

In addition to the natural simplicity offered by these algae, molds, and bacteria, many of them are cheap, convenient to grow and maintain in the laboratory, and easy to clone. Such advantages have made several of these creatures the organisms of choice for elucidating detailed mechanisms of chemical communication.

Obviously the compounds used as pheromones by these species must be chemically stable in water, but otherwise the chemical structures of the various pheromones have little in common. Perhaps surprisingly, these compounds do not have to be very soluble in water. Because pheromones are effective in such small amounts, a high concentration of the signal is not necessary. Only slight solubility is needed.

In addition to examining pheromones in some simple water organisms, we shall have an opportunity to say a bit about some of the instruments that chemists use in investigating pheromones. Also, we must speak briefly about what happens when a pheromone arrives at the recipient.

Sirenin, the Sex Attractant of a Water Mold

Allomyces, a microorganism usually called a water mold, grows on plant or animal debris in drains and ditches, along the edges of ponds, and in other moist, humble places. The life cycle of these water molds is intricate, involving both sexual and asexual reproduction.

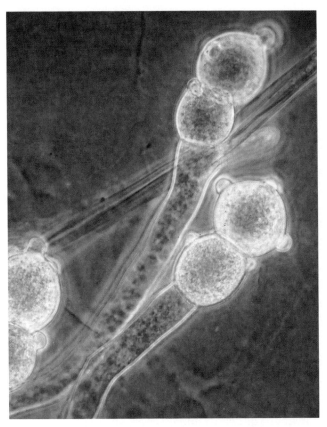

Male and female gametangia appear paired at the tips of these hyphae from *Allomyces*.

One phase of their existence consists of forms with male and female gametangia, which are small structures filled with gametes. When covered with water, the gametangia release the gametes through tiny pores in their walls. The male and female cells set free are destined to come together in pairs, fuse, and form a zygote, which is the first cell of a new individual, and which represents a new generation in the life cycle. The male gametes are highly mobile, the female gametes somewhat less so. They all move about in the water, each powered by the beating motion of a flagellum,

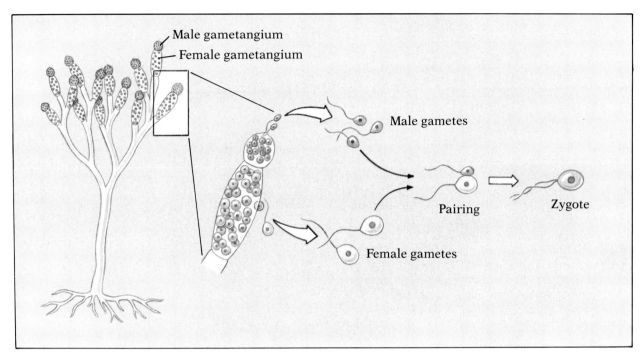

Sexual reproduction in the water mold *Allomyces*. Because the gametes swim freely in the water, their chances of pairing to form a zygote are much improved by the attractant released by the female cells.

which is a whiplike appendage, in this case a tail. Clearly, it is essential to the whole reproductive enterprise that a male gamete and female gamete find each other.

The meeting of the male and female gametes of *Allomyces* is not left simply to chance. Two or three minutes before leaving the gametangia, each large, colorless female gamete starts to release a pheromone known as sirenin. She discharges this substance into the water over the next six hours, and it is borne away from her by currents in the water and by motion of the pheromone molecules, spreading in a roughly regular fashion. As the molecules travel, they move farther away from one another, establishing a concentration gradient that points the way to the sender. The male gamete that picks up the signal some distance away can sense differences in the concentration of the pheromone and responds to the signal by swimming up the concentration gradient toward the source. Thus the pheromone lures the smaller, orange male cells to the female gamete so that fusion with one of them can take place. Other female gametes do not respond to sirenin.

There is some indication that the male cells also produce a pheromone, which attracts the female gametes. The active substance of the male pheromone has been paritally purified

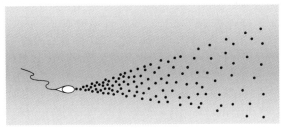

Direction of current ⟶

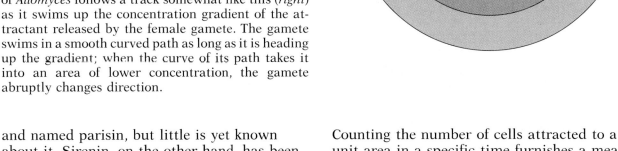

As molecules of a pheromone move away from their source (*left*), their random motion and the current spread them farther apart. The result is that the concentration of the pheromone in the water decreases as the distance from the source increases. A male gamete of *Allomyces* follows a track somewhat like this (*right*) as it swims up the concentration gradient of the attractant released by the female gamete. The gamete swims in a smooth curved path as long as it is heading up the gradient; when the curve of its path takes it into an area of lower concentration, the gamete abruptly changes direction.

and named parisin, but little is yet known about it. Sirenin, on the other hand, has been the object of extensive investigation.

In order to isolate and purify sirenin, scientists needed an effective bioassay. The male gametes will swim up a concentration gradient of sirenin toward its source, and the problem was how to turn this observation into a useful measure of the concentration of sirenin in a sample. The biologists solved this problem in the following way. Two solutions in a test chamber are separated by a semipermeable membrane. One is the solution to be tested for its content of the pheromone, and the other is a solution carrying a suspension of male gametes. These sperm cells are attracted by the pheromone, which diffuses slowly through the membrane, and they swim to the membrane and attach themselves to it in proportion to the concentration of sirenin on the other side.

Counting the number of cells attracted to a unit area in a specific time furnishes a measure of the concentration of sirenin in the test solution.

If this experiment is allowed to continue, the males are drawn to the membrane for about 90 minutes, and then they drift away. By this time, enough sirenin has diffused across the membrane to render the concentrations of the pheromone equal in the two solutions. After this, there is no net change with time and no concentration gradient on either side of the membrane. It is believed that the males detect this concentration gradient and move toward the source of the pheromone. Without a gradient, nothing prompts the males to swim to the membrane or remain there, and they simply wander off.

Another experiment has shown that the concentration of sirenin in a solution containing male gametes decreases with time. This indicates that the gametes metabolize the molecules of pheromone as they encounter them, either breaking them down or otherwise inactivating them. This metabolism of sirenin provides a way to get rid of the pheromone in the natural setting. It may be important for the sperm cell to destroy the pheromone after detection in order to continue perceiving the concentration gradient and to continue swimming toward the female gamete.

Scientists wished to determine how the male gametes detect a gradient in the sirenin concentration, and they considered two possible mechanisms, one spatial and the other temporal. To detect the gradient spatially, a gamete would require receptors at each end that would simultaneously sense and compare the local concentrations of pheromone to determine whether it was swimming up or down a gradient. To detect a gradient temporally, the swimming male cell would compare successive local concentrations of sirenin and then determine whether the concentration was increasing or decreasing with time. The behavior of male cells in a series of solutions in which the concentration of sirenin was either held constant or increased with time revealed that male *Allomyces* gametes monitor concentrations temporally. As the fertilization rate in this water mold is essentially 100 percent, temporal detection must work well.

In isolating sirenin chemists took advantage of the interesting observation that certain

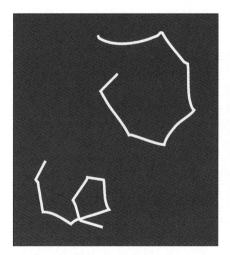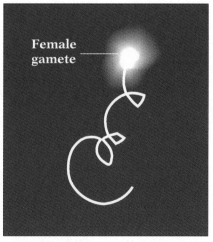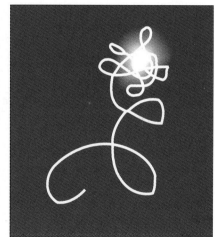

In the absence of sirenin (*left*), a male *Allomyces* gamete swims along short, smoothly arced paths interrupted by abrupt turns, giving the overall pathway a looping or spiral form. When a female gamete is nearby (*center*), the male swims smoothly up the concentration gradient, only pausing to adjust its path when the natural bend of its movement begins to take it away from the female. At close range (*right*), the male makes more frequent turns until a random hit brings it to the female. The longer runs and less frequent turns observed when the male gamete is exposed to a sudden, uniform increase in pheromone concentration are evidence that it uses a temporal sensing system.

strains of *Allomyces* produce either male or female gametes more than 95 percent of the time, rather than the mixture of the two typically formed in most strains. Sirenin is an effective attractant at a concentration of 24 picograms per milliliter of solution, so the female gametes synthesize and release only minute amounts of it. Large quantities of *Allomyces* were required for the isolation, and a strain that generates female gametes was grown up in five-gallon laboratory bottles. The scale of this operation was such that laboratory workers could process about 425 liters of solution containing female gametes and sirenin each week. After harvesting and processing of material, they finally produced 2.5 grams of sirenin to use in determining the pheromone's structure and in other studies.

Chemists elucidated the structure of sirenin by using a combination of chemical reactions and spectroscopic techniques that we shall discuss in the next section. Often after assigning a structure to a natural compound such as sirenin, chemists will synthesize this structure independently to provide a final check on their conclusions. In the process of synthesis, they build up a molecule with the assigned structure from simpler molecules by applying a sequence of chemical transformations in the laboratory. If laboratory tests prove the natural compound and the synthesized compound to be identical, this is good independent evidence that the assigned structure was indeed correct. For sirenin the final proof of structure rests on several independent syntheses.

Sometimes during such syntheses, related compounds become available. These may be chemical intermediates or side products encountered in the synthesis; sometimes they are molecules closely related to the target molecule. The synthesis of sirenin furnished several related compounds that were tested in the bioassay for their ability to attract the male gametes of *Allomyces*. All of these failed to elicit any response. Even small changes in the chemical structure of sirenin render its message unintelligible to the male gametes. We shall have more to say about the reasons for this sensitivity to structure in the following section on *Achlya*.

Steroids in Another Water Mold

Steroids are a group of compounds built on a skeleton of four rings of carbon atoms by attaching various functional groups and chains. These compounds have an ancient presence in living systems, and they occur in all types of organisms up and down the evolutionary scale, including bacteria and cyanobacteria. The most common steroid in nature is cholesterol, which is present in many animals and also in some plants. Among steroids there are a number of particularly important compounds that

Sirenin   2-Carene

Although sirenin was a previously unknown compound, its structure places it in a class of compounds that has been familiar to chemists for many years. A close relative is 2-carene, a long-known constituent of pine resins and pine oils. The heavy lines in the structure of sirenin indicate the portion of the molecular structure shared with 2-carene. The hexagon and the triangle in these structures represent rings of carbon atoms with attached hydrogens.

insects and vertebrates use as hormones. In vertebrates steroidal hormones include both the male sex hormone, testosterone, and the ovarian hormone, progesterone.

There is tremendous interest in how the molecules of steroid hormones function in carrying and delivering their various messages, owing to their central significance in human biology and medicine. In this regard *Achlya*, another water mold, has attracted some attention as a research organism because steroids regulate its sexual reproduction. *Achlya* produces two steroidal pheromones, one in male, and one in female individuals, or in some strains in the male and female portions of a single individual. Each pheromone is essential for the sexual development of the opposite sex. This dependence on steroids, along with the organism's relative biological simplicity and ease of maintenance in the laboratory, give *Achlya* some advantages as an organism for studying the details of how steroids work. The functions of steroids are unknown in most simple organisms, and they may or may not concern chemical communication. At present *Achyla* is unique in providing an unambiguous example of steroids serving as pheromones in a simple organism.

Under the microscope *Achlya* appears as a tangled mass of hollow threads or *hyphae*, each a few millimeters long. As these hyphae grow, they enlarge, lengthen, and branch, forming a collection of internally connected tubes, known as a *mycelium*. There are numerous nuclei and other intracellular structures in the completely interconnected hyphae, so that before the reproductive phase begins, a single mycelium can be regarded as one large cell.

Female mycelia of *Achlya* continuously produce a steroidal pheromone, antheridiol, and secrete it into the environment. Antheridiol takes its name from the male sex organs, antheridia, whose development it elicits. It acts upon nearby male mycelia, causing a certain growth reaction. Within one or two hours of receiving its message, male hyphae respond by forming antheridial branches off the main strands of the mycelium. These are tiny, sinuous extensions from the hyphae that begin to grow up the concentration gradient of the pheromone, advancing toward the female mycelium. As the antheridial branches are growing, antheridiol triggers a second response, and the male mycelium begins to secrete its own steroidal pheromone, oogoniol. This pheromone diffuses through the water and acts upon female mycelia, inducing them to initiate formation of female sex organs or oogonia. These appear as little polyplike growths off the female hyphae. Soon cross walls form, delimit-

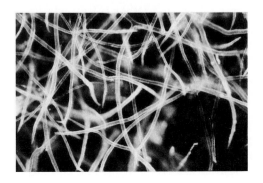
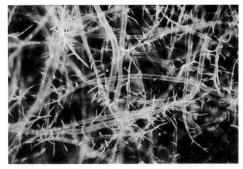

Male hyphae of the water mold *Achlya* (*left*) begin to form tiny antheridial branches (*right*) 1.5 hours after antheridiol is added to their environment.

ing the emerging oogonia from the main strands of the mycelium, and one to twenty egg cells develop in each oogonium.

The male antheridial branches have meanwhile continued their progress toward the female mycelium. The developing oogonia also appear to secrete antheridiol, because the antheridial branches seek out the oogonia and eventually become physically attached to their walls. Another response to antheridiol takes place at about this time. Cross walls divide off the tips of the antheridial branches and form antheridia, the fully formed male sex organs, in which sperm cells arise. The male antheridia are now attached to the walls of the female oogonia, and each structure holds its appropriate gametes. Next, a fertilization tube emerges from each antheridium and passes through the wall of an oogonium, connecting the male and female sex organs. The sperm pass from the antheridium, down this tube, and into the oogonium. There they unite with the egg cells to produce zygotes. Release of these zygotes from the oogonia completes the reproductive process, and under proper conditions, the zygotes germinate and develop into new individuals.

Very thorough biological experiments half a century ago demonstrated the operation of the two pheromones in *Achlya*, but chemical techniques for handling and determining the structures of complex substances in amounts as small as those available were lacking at the time. By the mid-1960s, techniques had improved, and T. C. McMorris and Alma Barksdale, both then at the New York Botanical Garden, undertook the isolation of the pheromone. For their work, the response of male mycelia to antheridiol provided a convenient bioassay. If a test solution induced formation of antheridial branches in 25 percent of the hyphae within 2 hours, the test was scored positive. Guided by this bioassay, fractionation finally provided about 2 milligrams of crystalline antheridiol from 85 liters of culture liquids of *Achlya*. Using the purified pheromone, investigators demonstrated that antheridiol elicits the growth of antheridial branches in male mycelia at concentrations as low as 10 picograms per milliliter.

To determine the structures of compounds like antheridiol, chemists often use standard spectroscopic techniques. Most spectroscopic techniques measure how much light a chemi-

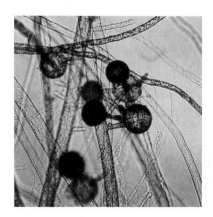 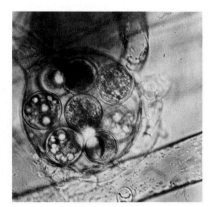

Sexual organs of the water mold *Achlya:* Female hyphae (*left*) with oogonia induced by the addition of the pheromone oogoniol; an oogonium containing eggs (*right*).

Ionization
chamber   Acceleration grids

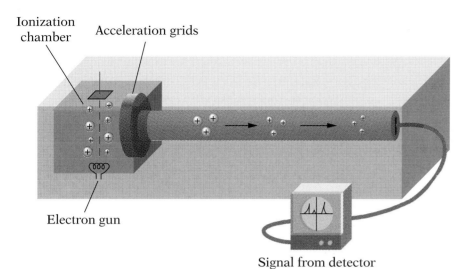

Electron gun

Signal from detector

Mass spectrometry is another physical technique that is widely used
in determining the structures of pheromones. In a mass spectrometer
a tiny amount of a compound is bombarded with high-energy electrons. This breaks the molecules up into ions of different sizes, and a
detector reports the size and relative abundance of these ions. From
this information a chemist can learn about the structure of the compound. In the particular kind of mass spectrometer shown, called a
time-of-flight mass spectrometer, ions are accelerated through a tube,
and those of different size move at different speed (the heaviest are
slowest). The detector judges the mass by the time of arrival.

cal compound absorbs. By "light" we mean
not only visible light but also ultraviolet, infrared, and related sorts of radiation. A device
called a spectrometer records how much of a
particular wavelength of light is absorbed by a
compound, producing a curve called a spectrum with peaks and valleys corresponding to
the absorption of more or less of the light.
These measurements require only a very small
amount of a compound and do not destroy it,
so the investigator can reuse the compound in
a later experiment. The absorption of light
reveals the presence and location of functional

groups and other structural features, and a
chemist can often write down the complete
three-dimensional structure of a molecule from
studying its spectra. Spectroscopic evidence
led to a proposed structure for antheridiol,
and this was then confirmed by two independent syntheses.

Using their knowledge of antheridiol's
structure, scientists were able to investigate
how the pheromone delivers its message. On
reaching the recipient organism, a pheromone
molecule, such as antheridiol, interacts with a
protein molecule known as a receptor. A recep-

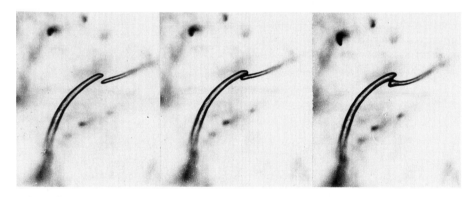

Antheridiol

tor has a chemical structure that permits it to interact with a specific compound or perhaps a few compounds of similar structure. These receptor and pheromone molecules can be thought of as a lock and key, and the key must properly fit the lock to work. The interaction of pheromone and receptor is the first step in the response of the recipient to the phero-

mone. Species from bacteria to mammals use protein receptors for detection of chemical signals.

Because of the particular biomedical importance of steroidal hormones for humans, the antheridiol receptor has been the object of considerable attention. Investigators have isolated this receptor and found that it is a sizeable protein, made from about 1,600 amino acids (the twenty different small molecules that are joined end to end to form proteins). The properties of the receptor molecule closely resemble those of steroidal hormone receptors from more complex organisms. Scientists have not isolated specific receptors for most of the pheromones we discuss, but they believe that these receptors exist and function in a generally similar fashion.

Oogoniol, the steroidal pheromone produced by male mycelia, presented a more diffi-

When the fungus *Mucor mucedo* reproduces sexually, erect hyphae of two mating types, (+) and (−), appear. Guided by the pheromone trisporic acid, two hyphae of different types grow toward each other until they make contact and fuse, eventually producing a new structure that will generate new individuals. The interesting feature of the process is that both mating types participate in the synthesis of the pheromone. Each type performs different steps in the synthesis, and the molecules undergoing transformation are passed back and forth (by diffusion through the water) until the synthesis of trisporic acid is complete.

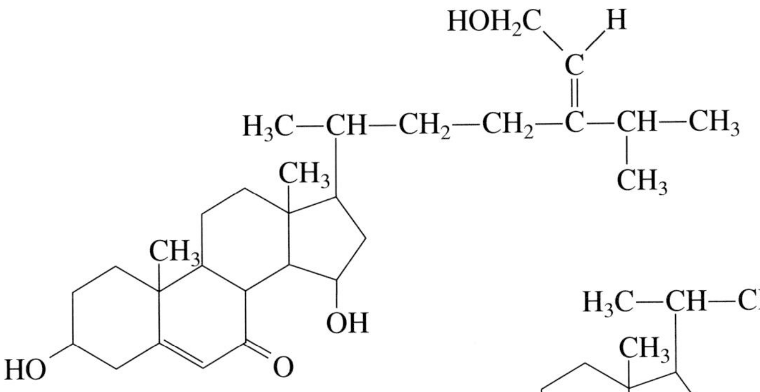

Dehydro-oogoniol

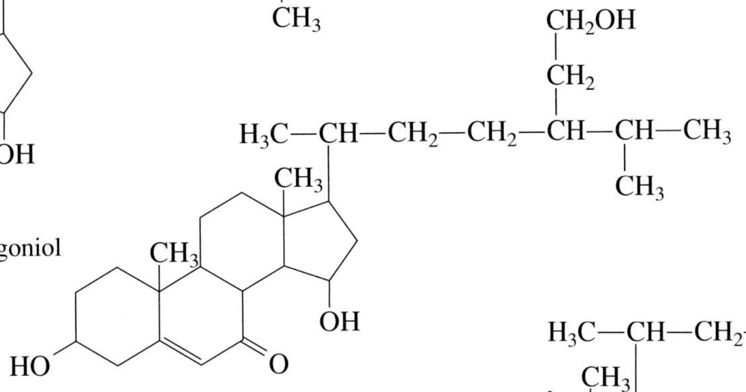

Oogoniol

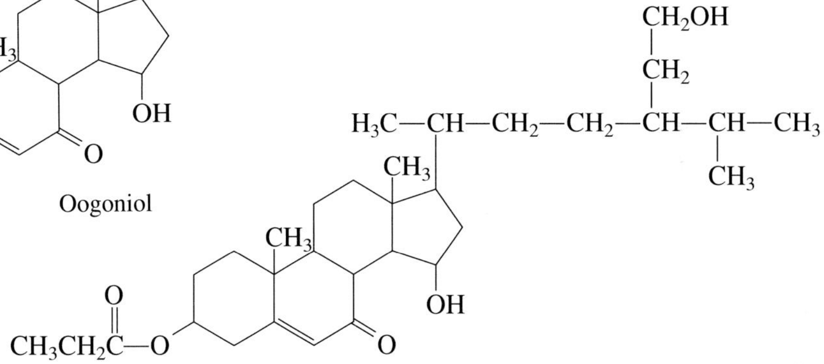

Propionic acid ester of oogoniol

cult chemical problem than did antheridiol. Male mycelia normally produce the pheromone only in response to stimulation by antheridiol, and it was difficult to induce formation of enough oogoniol to allow chemists to determine its structure. This obstacle was overcome when investigators discovered a strain of *Achlya heterosexualis* that secretes oogoniol without stimulation by antheridiol. From this strain the chemists could isolate useful amounts of the pheromone. (Another species of *Achlya, A. bisexualis,* had been the source for isolation of antheridiol.) The bioassay for oogoniol was analogous to the one used for antheridiol. Developing oogonia, which are easier to count than are antheridia, become visible after about 12 hours and reach a maximum after 24 to 48 hours.

As isolation and purification proceeded, a second obstacle arose. The pheromone turned out to be a mixture of several related substances. This made it more difficult to obtain pure compounds and to work out the structures, but finally the chemists recognized that the pheromonal mixture is based on two closely related steroids, oogoniol and dehydro-oogoniol. These compounds differ only by the presence in dehydro-oogoniol of a carbon-carbon double bond that is absent in oogoniol. (The name oogoniol was originally given to the natural pheromonal mixture before chemical structures were known, but it is now also the name used for one of the two steroids.) To complicate matters further, the steroids do not exist in the pheromone as such. Instead they are present as a mixture of *esters* with three simple carboxylic acids: acetic acid, propionic acid, and isobutyric acid.

Acetic acid   Propionic acid   Isobutyric acid

To form an ester, one hydroxyl (OH) group of the steroid molecule forms a bond with the carboxyl group of the acid. The drawing shows the steroids oogoniol and dehydro-oogoniol, and also the propionic acid ester of oogoniol as an example of the way the two steroids actually exist in the pheromone.

Although the components derived from dehydro-oogoniol are present in smaller amount, they are more significant biologically than those related to oogoniol. This is because they are about one hundred times more effective in inducing formation of oogonia, having this effect at concentrations as low as about 50 nanograms per milliliter. There has been no synthesis of any of the constituents of this pheromonal mixture, and with isolation from *Achlya* the only source, oogoniol remains in short supply.

Pheromones and Fragrance in Brown Algae

Brown algae are a quite diverse group, ranging in size from microscopic plants to giant kelps, which are huge golden-brown seaweeds that can be 50 meters (over 150 feet) long. Nearly all brown algae are marine organisms, living mostly along rocky shores in less than 15 meters of water and generally maintaining themselves by both sexual and asexual reproduction. In the course of their sexual reproduc-

tive cycle, female gametes are released into the water. The female gametes eventually settle down on the substrate and send out a pheromone that is attractive to the free-swimming male gametes. In some species the pheromone also brings about the release of male gametes from nearby individuals.

Over the past twenty years, the pheromones of some fifty species of brown algae have been investigated. Only ten different compounds seem to function as attractants in this large group, despite its considerable bio-

Fucus vesiculosus attractant

Typical pheromones of brown algae. Most contain only carbon and hydrogen, with eight or eleven carbon atoms and several carbon-carbon double bonds. Compounds of this sort are similar to gasoline or kerosene in their volatility and water solubility: they are moderately volatile and have low solubility in water. Like other properties we mentioned earlier, solubility depends on both molecular size and functional groups.

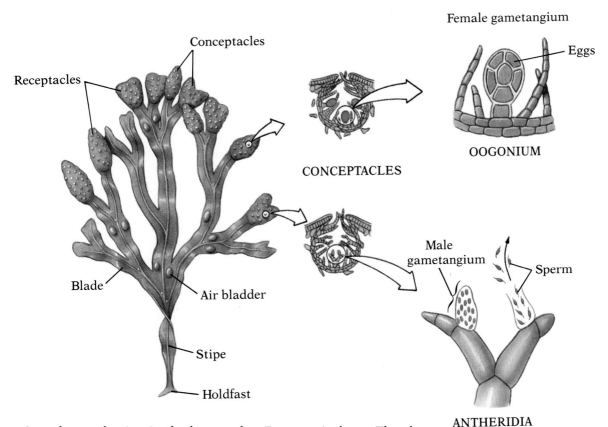

Sexual reproduction in the brown alga *Fucus vesiculosus.* The alga produces sperm and eggs in gametangia that are contained within small, dark, raised bodies called conceptacles, which are dotted across the surface of heart-shaped swellings called receptacles. This common green-brown seaweed is one to two feet long and is attached to rocks by the holdfast at its base. Its sexual attractant is a simple hydrocarbon having eight carbon atoms.

logical diversity. Most of these compounds are hydrocarbons, that is, they contain only atoms of carbon and hydrogen. In many cases several of these ten substances, along with other related compounds, are emitted by the female gametes of a single species, but only one of the group of compounds functions as a chemical signal for that species.

Several of the eleven-carbon pheromones, along with other similar substances, are also components of the essential oil of two Hawaiian brown algae, *Dictyopteris plagiogramma* and *Dictyopteris australis.* These fragrant sea-weeds wash up on Hawaiian beaches during heavy summer seas, and under the name limu lipoa they have a place in the local cuisine, chopped as a condiment for raw fish and other dishes. The hydrocarbons are responsible for the sweet odor of these seaweeds, but no one has shown that they act as pheromones in these two species.

Scientists had known of the attraction of sperm to egg in these algae since the 1940s, but the usual problems of collecting and identifying tiny amounts of material delayed structural work on the pheromones for many years. Isolation of the compounds was demanding. Even under laboratory conditions, the attainable concentrations of pheromone in the water were low, and scientists found it technically difficult to collect these volatile compounds from very dilute solution in seawater. In practice, they used a current of air to sweep the volatiles from solution and carry them to a

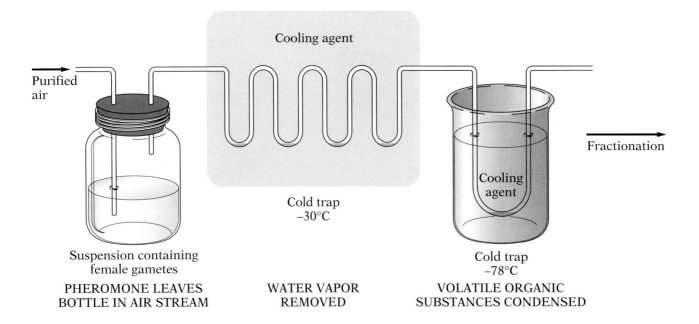

Purified air

Cooling agent

Cold trap −30°C

Cooling agent

Fractionation

Suspension containing female gametes

PHEROMONE LEAVES BOTTLE IN AIR STREAM

WATER VAPOR REMOVED

Cold trap −78°C

VOLATILE ORGANIC SUBSTANCES CONDENSED

To isolate the attractant pheromones of a brown alga, investigators placed a suspension of female gametes in seawater in a gas-washing bottle and then pumped dry purified air through the bottle at a rate of 25 milliliters per minute to sweep out the volatile substances, including the pheromones. The air stream emerging from the bottle passed into a cold trap at −30°C, a temperature low enough to freeze out most of the water vapor swept from the seawater with the pheromones but not low enough to freeze out the pheromones. Then the air stream was chilled to −78°C, and the volatile substances containing the pheromones condensed out and were collected in small U-tubes.

collector. Control experiments demonstrated that the efficiency of recovery was at best 17 percent and that it dropped rapidly as the volume of seawater being treated increased.

Investigators could collect only microgram amounts of volatile material from many brown algae, and often this small amount was a mixture of several very similar compounds. As a rule, it was not feasible to fractionate these minute samples or to carry out bioassays in the usual manner. Instead, the scientists separated microgram or nanogram amounts of these mixtures into their components by passing them through an instrument called a gas chromatograph, from which each component emerged at a separate time. By passing the chromatograph's output stream directly into a mass spectrometer, they were able to record the mass spectrum separately for each component without ever handling the components individually. For molecules as simple as these ten pheromones, these limited measurements restricted the likely structures in each case to a few possibilities, but often did not permit a final choice. For example, distinguishing between Z and E carbon-carbon double bonds was usually impossible. In proving the structures of the pheromones of brown algae, chemists independently synthesized the several candidate structures suggested by the spectra for each compound. By comparing the spectra and biological properties of the synthetic candidate compounds with those of each natural substance, the scientists narrowed down the possibilities and assigned a structure to each pheromone.

The low water-solubility and high volatility of these pheromones required novel bioassays. For a qualitative indication of attractivity, investigators adsorbed the test compound on minute particles of silica and then placed these particles in water containing male gametes. They could assess visually the effectiveness of these particles in drawing male cells to their surfaces. In a more quantitative approach, the investigators dissolved the test compound in a dense oil which was then dispersed in water as a suspension of droplets less than 1 millimeter in diameter. The oil itself was inert, that is, it would not react chemically with the pheromones or interfere with the response of the male gametes. Within a few minutes, male gametes were attracted to the microdroplets if they carried an active pheromone, and dark-field photomicrographs provided a permanent record of the density of gametes at individual droplets. The investigators obtained a semiquantitative estimate of the attractivity of the test compound from a statistical treatment of the counts of male gametes per droplet recorded in the photomicrographs.

One of the factors controlling the amount of each test substance reaching the male cells in this bioassay is its relative solubility in the carrier oil droplet and in the surrounding water. This property is ordinarily expressed as a ratio of the two solubilities involved, and this ratio is called a partition coefficient. Partition coefficients between seawater and the carrier oil differ over one hundred-fold for the various compounds being tested. For this reason, to make accurate comparisons of the attractivity of these compounds, the investigators had to measure and take into consideration the partition coefficient for each compound.

With this bioassay investigators could determine the threshold concentrations of pheromone needed to elicit the response of male gametes. In the most sensitive species examined, the male gamete responded when interacting with no more than 1,250 molecules of pheromone per second. This may seem like rapid bombardment of the gamete by the pheromone, but molecules are not like bullets.

Dieter Müller at the University of
Konstanz developed this bioassay for
sex attractants of brown algae. Each
circle contains a small drop of water
in which microdroplets of oil are dispersed. The oil in (B), (C), and (D) contains identical concentrations of one
of the purified pheromones; the oil in
(A) contains no pheromone and serves
as the control. After preparing the
four drops, the investigator adds
male gametes to each drop of water
and disperses them evenly. He waits
4 minutes and then makes a photomicrograph recording the distribution
of the gametes. By counting the cells
in a standard area [see (D)] in the
photomicrograph, the investigator
can estimate attractivity. The bar at
the right is 1 millimeter long and indicates the scale of the experiment.

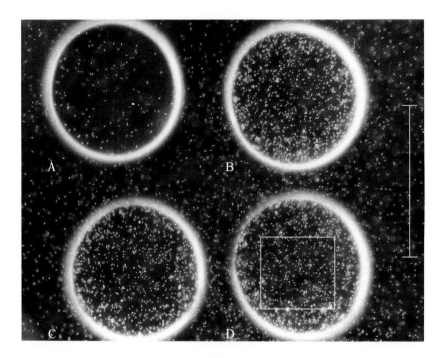

On the molecular level it is really a trivial
number of encounters, because molecular interactions usually involve astronomical numbers of particles. For comparison, a spherical
object about the size of a male gamete (several
micrometers in diameter) in the air under ordinary conditions of temperature and pressure
is struck by about 5×10^{23} molecules of air
gases per second. On this scale, 1,250 is totally
negligible.

Scientists do not yet understand the male
cell's reception and internal transmission of
the signal provided by these pheromone molecules, but the resulting cellular motion, the
swimming toward the female cell, has been
studied in the gametes of several brown algae,
and also in *Allomyces*. Swimming patterns and
cell shape differ among the species studied.

In the species of brown algae most thoroughly examined in this regard, *Ectocarpus*

siliculosus, the male gametes are pear-shaped
cells, about 7 to 8 micrometers long, and fitted
with two asymmetrically placed flagella, one
in front and one in the rear. The front flagellum is flexible, and the rear flagellum is rigid.
Until he detects the pheromone, the male cell
moves along a straight line, holding his rear
flagellum straight back and beating his front
flagellum up and down with an irregular
rhythm. On detecting the pheromone, the male
cell begins to swim in a clockwise loop. He
does this by setting the rear flagellum at an
angle to his cell body, so that it serves as a
rudder, and then beating it rapidly. Whether
swimming straight ahead or in loops, the male
speeds along at 100 to 140 micrometers (some
twelve to twenty body lengths) per second. As
he proceeds up the gradient and the pheromone concentration rises, the angle of the rudder increases and his loops become tighter and

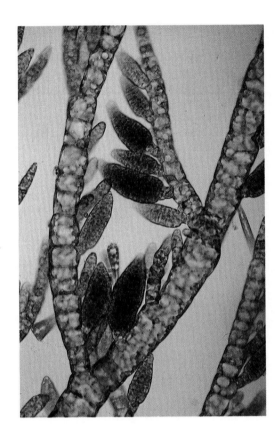

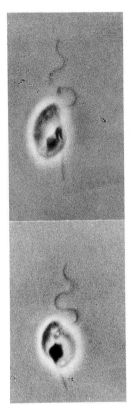

Ectocarpus siliculosus is a filamentous alga, formed of many thin branched strands. In a microscopic view of filaments (*left*), the dark shapes extending from the filament branches are gametangia. Male gametes of *Ectocarpus* (*right*) have a long flexible flagellum in front and a short rigid flagellum in the rear.

tighter. He approaches the female cell, describing ever smaller encircling loops. Finally the two cells touch, their membranes unite, and they fuse.

Pheromones in a Common Bacterium

We should mention finally what is probably the most complete study of pheromones in a simple microorganism. *Streptomyces faecalis* is a common bacterium that is found in the intestinal tract and feces of most mammals and birds, including man. It is also an important

pathogen, and in man it leads to infection of the urinary tract, infection of wounds, and sometimes to inflammation of the heart. *S. faecalis* is exceptionally hardy and thrives under extremes of temperature and salinity that most bacteria cannot endure.

As with other bacteria, two cells of *S. faecalis* can come together in conjugation for the transfer of DNA from one cell to the other. This mating process requires the presence of an "aggregation substance" on the surface of one cell and a "binding substance" on the surface of the other. With both substances present, the two cells will stick together if they collide, and conjugation can take place.

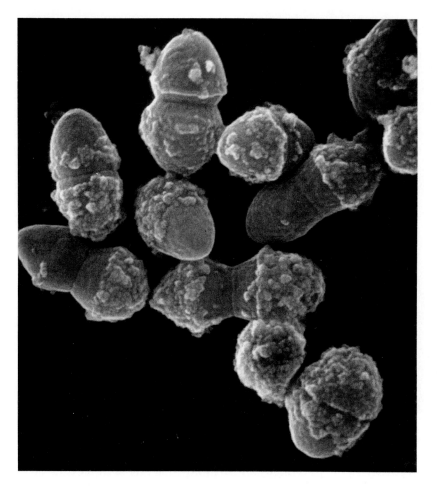

Cells of the bacterium *Streptomyces faecalis* clump together after exposure to an aggregation pheromone. Adsorbed gold particles make the aggregation substance on the surface of each cell clearly visible in this photomicrograph produced by Dr. Reinhard Wirth of the University of Munich.

Over the past decade and more, Don B. Clewell and his research group at the University of Michigan have explored mating in *S. faecalis*. As a result, we now understand a good deal about the genetic and molecular events involved. There is more than academic interest here. Conjugation is thought to enhance the spread of resistance of *S. faecalis* to antibiotics, and in a microbe responsible for human disease, resistance to antibiotics is a practical medical matter. Very briefly put, the aggregation substance develops on one cell surface in response to one of several compounds released by another cell; these compounds are all peptides, short strings of amino acids bonded together. These peptides are thus sex pheromones with an important role. Two of these pheromones have been identified as peptides of similar structure, each containing eight amino acids. It seems likely that analogous pheromonal systems exist in other bacteria.

These examples demonstrate that relatively simple organisms make substantial use of chemical communication in their lives, mostly as sex attractants between their gametes and as carriers of other signals important in reproduction. In more complex lives pheromones can also carry many other sorts of messages that are vital to success, as we see in the next chapter when we consider pheromones among the invertebrates.

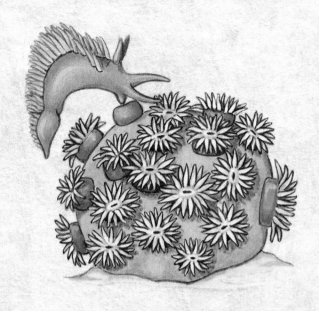

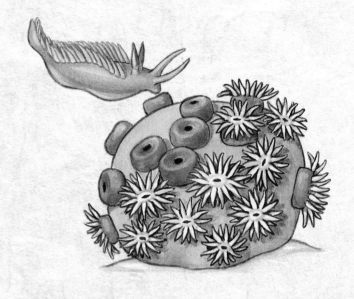

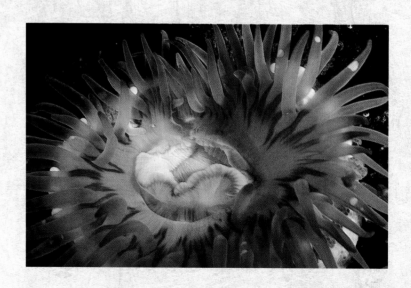

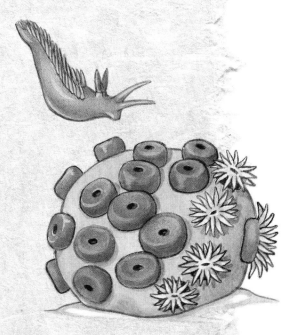

3

ALARMS AND ALLUREMENTS

■ When the sea anemone *Anthopleura elegantissima* is attacked by a sea slug, it quickly draws in its tentacles, closes its mouth, and releases an alarm pheromone. This waterborne signal spreads through the dense colony of anemones, and each individual closes as the warning reaches it.

*I*nvertebrates are animals that have no backbones. They form a huge and incredibly diverse group; from spiders to starfish; from butterflies to sponges, ticks, clams, tapeworms, and lobsters; from giant squids more than 15 meters long to mites that live in the ears of moths. About 95 percent of the recognized living animal species are invertebrates, and they occupy every conceivable environment and ecological niche that supports life. Eight or ten thousand new species are described each year. Chemical communication is as important here as it is anywhere, and the pheromones of these creatures will occupy our attention for the next two chapters.

In some of the simple organisms discussed earlier, attractant pheromones brought free-swimming gametes together in water for what is called external fertilization. Attractant pheromones are also important for many invertebrates, where they more frequently bring together two organisms rather than two gametes. Invertebrates provide examples of external fertilization, but fertilization is internal in many of these creatures. In most cases there is relatively little information about the chemistry of these attractants, but most of the ones that have been examined at all appear to be peptides or proteins.

These animals use pheromones not only as attractants but for numerous other purposes as well, as might be expected since the lives of most invertebrates are more complex than those of algae and fungi. There are pheromones that influence aspects of reproduction other than attraction. There are alarm pheromones that prompt organisms to evacuate an area rapidly or, if they are sedentary, to assume appropriate defense postures. There are aggregation pheromones that bring members of a species together, in some cases guiding juvenile forms to an established adult habitat.

$$\underset{\begin{array}{c}|\\CH_3\end{array}}{\overset{\begin{array}{c}H\\|\end{array}}{H_2N-C-COOH}}$$

An amino acid

$$\underset{\begin{array}{cc}|&|\\CH_3&H\end{array}}{\overset{\begin{array}{cc}H&H\\|&|\end{array}}{H_2N-C-CONH-C-COOH}}$$

A typical dipeptide (two amino acids)

Peptides, like proteins, are derived from amino acids. The distinction between them is one of size. Peptides consist of two to twenty or thirty amino acid units. Larger molecules are usually called proteins.

There are trail pheromones that permit one individual to make paths for others to follow, and there are other signals that provoke aggressive behavior.

Behavioral evidence for pheromones is widespread among the invertebrates, although there are few extensive studies of their chemistry and biology. One of the most fundamental findings is that chemical communication is used by many different kinds of organisms. Despite their widely varying habitats, ways of life, and physical forms, all sorts of invertebrates send chemical signals to other members of their species. In this chapter we look at pheromones in some of these creatures. About half of the invertebrates are insects, and this large group will be discussed separately in the next chapter.

Sending an Alarm

The sea anemone *Anthopleura elegantissima* produces one of the chemically best investigated invertebrate pheromones. Sea anemones are in the group called cnidarians or coelenterates, which also includes such creatures as Portuguese men-of-war, jellyfishes, and corals. As adults, many sea anemones are brightly colored, and they grow like pretty flowers attached to rocks in coastal waters throughout the world. Structurally, they consist of a vertical, cylindrical column, closed at one end by a base, which fastens the organism to a rock. The open upper end of the cylinder forms a mouth that the anemone can draw closed by pursestring-like muscles. This mouth is surrounded by tentacles, and when anemones are feeding, the mouth is open and visible. The tentacles wave about, locating food and forcing it into the mouth, in many species after paralyzing it with a toxin. Some robust species can even handle small fish in this way.

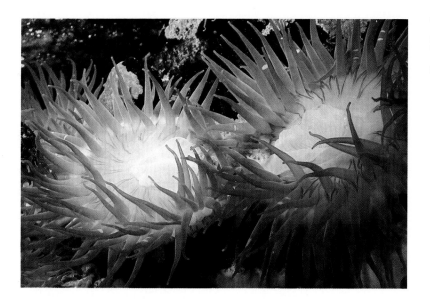

Through longitudinal division one sea anemone *Anthopleura elegantissima* has become two individuals, which are now almost completely separated.

Although they appear to be firmly fixed to the rocky substrate, anemones can actually glide along on their bases by waves of muscular contraction. A few species are able to swim or burrow into muddy bottoms.

Anthopleura elegantissima is a common sea anemone about 2 centimeters (0.8 inch) in diameter that decorates intertidal rocks along the California coast. If it is wounded, this animal produces an alarm pheromone that warns neighboring members of its species. On receiving this signal, an anemone undergoes a rapid convulsion unlike that produced by any other stimulus. First it gives a series of quick, convulsive flexures of its tentacles toward the base of the column; then the tentacles withdraw into the mouth cavity, and the mouth closes tightly. All of this happens in less than 3 seconds. If the alarm signal does not persist, the anemone resumes normal behavior within 2 hours.

Working with specimens of *A. elegantissima* gathered from intertidal rocks in Monte-rey, California, Nathan Howe at the Hopkins Marine Station of Stanford University investigated the chemistry and biology of this pheromone. In laboratory experiments Howe set groups of anemones, one group after another, in a flowing stream of water. He then wounded an anemone at the upper end of the stream. First, anemones near the wounded animal contracted, and then each group downstream reacted sequentially as the flowing water carrying the pheromone reached it. This rapid alarm reaction provided the basis of a sensitive bioassay for work with the pheromone. Using the bioassay as a guide, Howe isolated colorless needlelike crystals from homogenized sea anemones. Spectroscopic studies yielded the structure of this compound, which Howe named anthopleurine. This is an exceptional pheromone in that it is an ionic compound: it has a positive and a negative ion that are not joined together by a chemical bond. The positive ion is made up of many atoms, and this is the active part of the com-

$$Cl^-$$

$$H_3C-^+N-CH_2-\underset{|}{\overset{|}{CH}}-\underset{|}{\overset{|}{CH}}-COOH$$

with CH₃ groups on the nitrogen and OH groups on the carbons:

$$\begin{array}{c} CH_3 \\ | \\ H_3C-^+N-CH_2-CH-CH-COOH \\ | \qquad | \quad | \\ CH_3 \quad OH \; OH \end{array}$$

Anthopleurine

pound. That is, it is the positive ion of anthopleurine that interacts with the receptor
molecule in the recipient anemone. Anthopleurine can trigger the alarm response at a
concentration of 74 picograms per milliliter of
seawater.

Ordinarily, *A. elegantissima* lives in rather
turbulent waters. The endless movement rapidly disperses and dilutes anthopleurine as it
is released, so the pheromone has limited effect, despite its high biological activity. It can
alert other sea anemones to impending danger
only if they are within a few centimeters of

the wounded individual that issues the warning. This limited range is still helpful, because
A. elegantissima often forms densely packed
colonies. It commonly reproduces asexually
simply by dividing in two longitudinally, eventually creating a cluster of individuals.

However, *A. elegantissima* also has a much
more effective means of disseminating its
warning signal. It uses one of its most persistent predators to deliver anthopleurine to
endangered anemones, and it is this curious
defense that makes this anemone particularly
interesting. The predator is *Aeolidia papillosa*,
a carnivorous marine slug that may grow to
be 2 or 3 centimeters long. Its favorite food is
A. elegantissima, and the two species are often
found together. Anthopleurine is present
throughout the body of *A. elegantissima*, and
when *A. papillosa* feeds on the anemone, it ingests a considerable amount of the pheromone.
The slug does not metabolize anthopleurine
readily but stores the pheromone in its tissues.

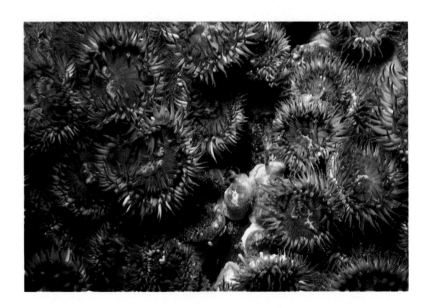

A small gap separates two crowded, genetically different colonies of the sea
anemone *Anthopleura elegantissima*.

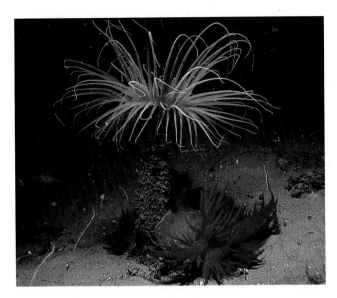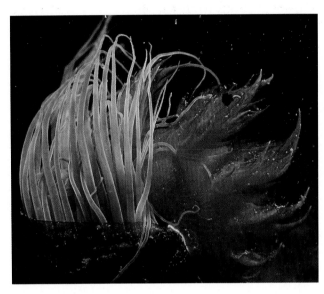

A sea slug attacking a different species of sea anemone. The slug crawls up the vertical column of the sea anemone to reach the tentacles that it feeds on.

From there anthopleurine is released slowly into the water, and for at least five days after feeding on *A. elegantissima*, the slug sets off the alarm reaction in anemones whenever it approaches them.

The slug prefers to nibble on tentacles, but in assaulting a forewarned anemone that has withdrawn its tentacles and closed its mouth, the slug is reduced to attacking the base or column of the organism. The concentration of anthopleurine happens to be much higher in these tissues than in the tentacles, so that in attacking an alerted anemone the slug gets a comparatively large dose of the pheromone. *A. papillosa* pays a price for its meal, and the old conundrum "Who will bell the cat?" finds a simple answer here. In consuming a bit of the anemone, the slug turns itself into an early-warning device that proclaims its threat to anemones wherever it goes.

Attracting a Mate

Roundworms, or nematodes, are everywhere. A spadeful of garden soil can contain millions of them. These are slender worms with unsegmented bodies that generally have a smooth and shiny surface. They come in lengths from less than a millimeter (0.04 inch) to 8 meters (26 feet). Many sorts of nematodes are free living, but they have also parasitized virtually every kind of plant and animal.

These are the worms responsible for hookworm in the old South, pinworm in children, heartworm in dogs, and a host of other maladies. Both Aristotle and Hippocrates mention nematodes, and in Egyptian sources there are even earlier references to them as scourges of mankind. They lead us to eat well-cooked pork to avoid trichinosis, which is a sometimes fatal disease that follows infestation by *Trichi-*

nella spiralis. This nematode is common in pigs, and a human who eats meat from an infected animal can acquire the disease. The infection often has only mild effects and goes unnoticed by the host, but evidence from autopsy records indicates that nearly 20 percent of the population of the United States has suffered from trichinosis at some time. About fifty other species of nematodes also live in humans. Fortunately, most of these parasites lead quiet lives and have no serious overt effects on their hosts.

Other nematodes parasitize plants and are responsible for significant damage to crops. There are about seventy-five species of cyst nematodes that attack the roots of agricultural plants throughout the world, causing substantial losses in crops of soybeans, potatoes, sugarbeets, grains, and grasses. Certain nematodes also carry viruses that cause other plant diseases. A better understanding of the biology of these pests, including their use of chemical signals, could lead to better strategies for their control. For this reason pheromones in these plant parasites attract serious attention from agricultural scientists.

Intensive studies of pheromones in nematodes began in the 1960s. There is good behavioral evidence in several species for a chemical attractant in one sex or the other, but the first complete identification of a nematode pheromone came only in 1989. The creature producing this signal is the soybean cyst nematode *Heterodera glycines*, which is a serious agricultural problem in many parts of the world. This tiny worm attacks the growing root tips of the soybean plant (*Glycine max*) and other legumes. The female worm emits a pheromone that attracts males and also causes them to display a distinctive coiling behavior. The significance of this coiling is uncertain, but it led to the development of a convenient bioassay.

Earlier efforts to identify this pheromone had not been successful. As you have probably realized by now, the quality of the bioassay is critical in the isolation of biologically active

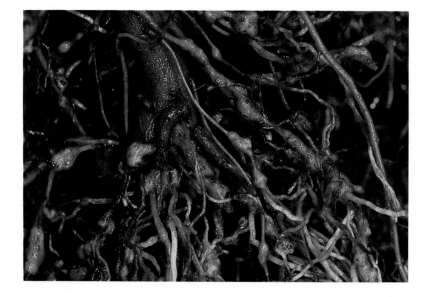

The swellings or galls on these cotton roots are caused by an infestation of the root-knot nematode *Meloidogyne incognita.* This economically important pest attacks a variety of other crops, including tobacco and tomato.

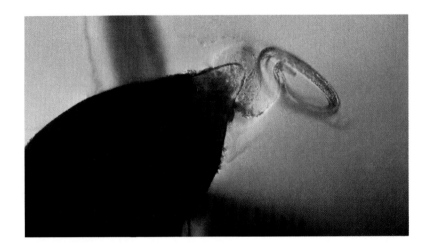

A small male soybean cyst nematode appears coiled at the posterior end of a much larger bloated female. The female's head is buried in the vertical soybean root seen in the background.

compounds. Robin N. Huettel and her coworkers at the Agricultural Research Service laboratories of the United States Department of Agriculture succeeded in isolating and identifying this pheromone following their development of a bioassay that was both quick and efficient. The procedure depended on a rapid, reliable response that could be assessed in a small number of males. Huettel and her coworkers placed male worms in water in groups of ten and aerated them to remove any traces of the natural attractant pheromone. They then transferred the males to a tiny, measured droplet of test solution on a plate, left them for 30 seconds, and examined them under a stereomicroscope. The observer could immediately count the number of worms displaying the coiling reaction, and this provided a semiquantitative measure of the pheromone in the test solution. Using this bioassay, Huettel's team could rapidly screen the material initially extracted from female worms and then continue to follow the purification of the pheromone.

Isolation of the pheromone required large numbers of female nematodes. The work began with the removal by hand of 10-to-12-day-old females in batches of one thousand from soybean root tips. A crude extract of 23,870 females provided the biologically active starting material for chemical purification. With the new bioassay as a guide, fractionation of this material finally yielded 315 nanograms of a pure compound that had all the properties of the pheromone. Spectroscopic data suggested that this compound was vanillic acid, and comparison with an authentic sample of that compound showed this assignment to be correct. Authentic vanillic acid has the same spectroscopic properties as the material isolated from *H. glycines*, it produces the same coiling response in the bioassay as the natural pheromone, and it serves equally well as an attractant for the male. A droplet containing about 350 picograms of vanillic acid reproducibly provokes the coiling response in about 60 percent of the males tested. At concentrations more than one hundred times higher, well above the natural level, it induces a paralysis-like effect in the males.

Vanillic acid is one of several compounds that are ubiquitous in the natural world as

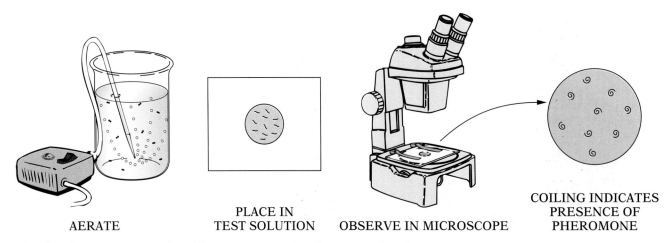

AERATE   PLACE IN   OBSERVE IN MICROSCOPE   COILING INDICATES
                TEST SOLUTION   PRESENCE OF
                                                              PHEROMONE

For their bioassay, Huettel and her team aerated male nematodes: the movement of the water produced by the air bubbles should have washed off any natural attractant adhering to the worms. They then placed groups of ten males in a test solution containing fractions of the female extract, and counted the number of males displaying the coiling reaction.

products of the breakdown of woody material by fungi. The rotting of a fallen tree on the forest floor is largely the consequence of fungal metabolism of the dead wood, and one of the waste products formed in this universal process is vanillic acid. Wherever wood rots, a small amount of vanillic acid is left behind in the soil. In view of this wide distribution, it was important to establish that the sample of

vanillic acid isolated as a pheromone in *H. glycines* indeed originated in the extracted nematodes and did not come from the soybean plants or the soil or some other extraneous source. Control experiments demonstrated that none of these other materials contained vanillic acid, and this confirmed that the material isolated did originate in the female nematode. You may wonder why, if vanillic acid is so

Vanillic acid takes its name from vanillin. As you can see, the two are structurally identical, except that vanillic acid is a carboxylic acid, and vanillin is what is called an aldehyde. Vanillin is the principal component of vanilla extract and the main flavor ingredient of the vanilla bean.

Vanillic acid   Vanillin

common in the soil, the *H. glycines* males are not confused by it. The answer probably is that the concentration of vanillic acid in soil is generally too low to be effective as a pheromone.

In the United States the farmer's primary defense against soybean predation by *H. glycines* is the planting of resistant strains, and this is not a wholly satisfactory strategy. Identification of the pheromonal attractant in *H. glycines* may lead to new techniques for protection of the soybean crop. As the Agricultural Research Service investigators commented in their account, " . . . we are hopeful the report here of the determination of the first structure of a compound with sex pheromone activity in nematodes might lead to development of future novel and environmentally safe control strategies for these pests."

An Earthworm's Alarm

There are several groups of distinctive wormlike creatures among the invertebrates, but to many people "worm" ordinarily means earthworm. This is the worm that the early bird is supposed to get, and more importantly, it is the worm that is indispensable for keeping the soil of farm and forest in good condition. Earthworms bring topsoil to the surface by the ton through their burrowing and eating. Charles Darwin noted that all topsoil passes through their bodies every few years and declared that "it may be doubted if there are any other animals which have played such an important part in the history of the world as these lowly organized creatures."

The common earthworm *Lumbricus terrestris* secretes a mucus over its full length. This mucus serves as a lubricant as the worm moves through its burrow, and it may also bind dirt particles together and prevent collapse of the burrow walls. If a worm is stressed with a pinch or an electrical shock, it begins to secrete much more mucus and adds an alarm pheromone to the secretion. Other earthworms find the mucus from stressed worms repulsive: worms placed on a glass plate that carries a drop of this mucus quickly wriggle off the plate, whereas they ignore mucus from unstressed worms.

Mucus from stressed worms has two other noteworthy properties. At least four diverse vertebrate species that ordinarily eat earthworms found this mucus offensive in behavioral experiments. A spotted salamander (*Ambystoma maculatum*) pushed a mucus-covered worm from its mouth and made grooming movements to clean the mucus away. A group of bobwhite quail (*Colinus virginianus*) pecked at stressed worms and then wiped their beaks on the bottom of their cages. Grasshopper mice (*Onychomyns leucogaster*) and American toads (*Bufo americanus*) also tried and rejected stressed worms. None of these predators would eat earthworms that had been stressed, although they quickly devoured unstressed worms. On the other hand, red-sided garter snakes (*Thamnophis sirtalis parietalis*), which also regularly consume earthworms, were attracted to mucus from stressed worms. How many different compounds are responsible for these various responses? We know that the garter snake attractant is a protein and that the alarm substance is a smaller molecule. Earthworm predators that reject stressed worms may be responding to other components of the secretion. These details remain to be worked out, but it is clear that the earthworm has an effective defensive strategy that warns other worms of danger and repels certain predators. The garter snake seems to have turned this defensive secretion to its own advantage.

A Trail to Follow,
An Alarm to Heed

The mollusks form a large group whose best-known members are clams, oysters, octopuses, and snails. They provide more food for man than any other group of invertebrates. The group also includes slugs that live on land and in water, some having shells resembling those of snails, and some with shells much reduced or nonexistent. The sea slug *Navanax inermis* is an ornately colored, soft-bodied, hermaphroditic creature, some 5 to 15 centimeters (2 to 6 inches) long, that lives in shallow subtidal habitats along the Pacific coast from northern California to southern Baja California.

Like other slugs and the earthworm, *N. inermis* lubricates its way with a mucus secretion as it slides along the bottom. Experiments with various sea slugs have shown that the mucus trails secreted during ordinary movement contain a trail pheromone and that a second slug can follow such a path very efficiently. For *N. inermis*, pursuing trails of its own and other species is not an idle pastime but an enterprise critical to finding both food and mates. *N. inermis* is a voracious predator on other slugs and is also cannibalistic. There

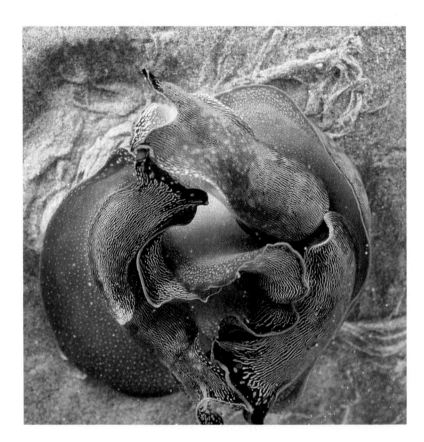

Two specimens of the sea slug *Navanax inermis* mating.

is no sense of direction in its tracking, however, so often it will faithfully follow a trail away from, rather than toward, the source.

There is yet no chemical information about this trail pheromone, but a second signal from the mucus has been thoroughly investigated. If *N. inermis* is attacked or molested, it begins to secrete into the slime trail a bright yellow material that can persist on the bottom for several hours. Another slug following the trail and encountering this yellow material responds by turning sharply from the trail and retreating. The yellow material thus is an alarm pheromone. It is secreted directly into the mucus trail from a gland located on the underside of the animal. Anatomists had previously described this structure and named it the "yellow gland," but its function had remained obscure. This yellow alarm pheromone aroused the curiosity and interest of Howard L. Sleeper, Valerie J. Paul, and William Fenical at the Scripps Institution of Oceanography, and they proceeded to isolate it and examine it in detail.

N. inermis will secrete 3 to 5 milligrams of the yellow alarm pheromone in response to a pinch on the back with a pair of tweezers. This made the material readily available to the Scripps investigators for chemical identification and biological studies. Purification of the secretion finally yielded three major components of the pheromone, which were identified and named navenones A, B, and C. The color of each of the navenones is an intense yellow, which turns out to be biologically significant, as will be explained.

The highly reproducible trail-following behavior of *N. inermis* offered a suitable bioassay for guiding fractionation of the alarm pheromone and for determining the pheromonal activity of the purified navenones. To establish a standard behavior pattern for use in the bioassay, a fresh specimen of the slug was

Navenone A

Navenone B

Navenone C

The system of double bonds present in the navenones causes them to be bright yellow.

allowed to wander freely in a laboratory aquarium with a bottom of white sand, until it had travelled about a meter and had deposited an elaborate slime trail with at least two acute turns. The normal mucus secretion is colorless, so the investigator deposited blue grains of sand behind the meandering slug to mark the track. Then the investigator sharply pinched the animal on its back. It reacted by contracting severely then resumed its crawling, now secreting the alarm pheromone into its trail, making it easily visible against the white sand. At this point the investigator carefully removed the first slug from the aquarium and introduced a second specimen at the start of the freshly laid trail. This second slug immediately began to follow the trail, but when it arrived at the alarm pheromone, it turned off the trail abruptly. The second slug then searched until it encountered a portion of trail free of alarm pheromone and began following it. Often in its search, the slug chanced upon its own earlier track while travelling in the opposite direction. It then faithfully traced this trail back to the starting point. When the alarm pheromone was artificially introduced into the colorless trail left by the first slug, the second slug showed the same behavior. In both cases, 90 to 95 percent of the time the second animal left the trail on reaching the alarm substance. The individual navenones, purified from the secretion and added to the trail, had the same effect. All the natural components of the pheromone are active above a lower limit of about 2 micrograms per milliliter of *N. inermis* slime.

Owing directly to their yellow color, the navenones absorb sunlight, and they are chemically unstable when light shines on them in seawater. The yellow pheromone deposited in a mucus track along the shallow sea bottom fades in the sunlight and is bleached away in a few daylight hours. The sensitivity of the navenones to light thus provides a mechanism for their removal from the environment. Timely termination of a warning signal is desirable, because the warning transmitted by an alarm pheromone is useless or possibly even counterproductive once the cause for alarm has passed. On land, alarm substances can be rapidly dispersed and diluted by diffusion and wind currents, and signals released directly into water are similarly dissipated in short order. The alarm pheromone of *N. inermis*, however, is not readily diluted or washed away by seawater but remains suspended and protected in the slime track on the bottom. Without degradation through the action of sunlight, it might remain active for days. Sunshine obliterates the yellow warning message after a reasonable length of time.

A Hatching Pheromone: A Mother Signals Her Embryos

Crustaceans are a class of the arthropods, the largest animal group. The most familiar crustaceans are shrimps, lobsters, crabs, and barnacles, but the class includes thousands of other kinds of creatures, most of which live in water. A crustacean whose behavior has been well studied is the arctic barnacle *Balanus balanoides*, whose range extends as far south as the estuaries of Cornwall and Brittany. Owing to persistent efforts for more than a quarter century by D. J. Crisp of the Marine Science Laboratories in North Wales (United Kingdom), we have an unusually detailed picture of pheromonal activity in this barnacle. At least two different chemical signals from the adult barnacle govern activities of the larvae.

After the female lays a mass of fertilized eggs, she holds then in her mantle cavity during their development. This cavity is a space within the barnacle that is in direct communication with the sea. Experiments in the laboratory have shown that developed eggs hatch into larvae only after the females carrying them are fed. Arctic waters are not rich in foodstuffs year round, it is undoubtedly advantageous to release the larvae only when food is available for them. In nature the eggs of *B. balanoides* hatch just at the time of the spring algal bloom, when there is plenty of food for both adults and larvae. Extensive studies have demonstrated that feeding prompts the female barnacle to release a hatching pheromone into her mantle cavity where it comes into contact with the developing eggs. This pheromone acts directly on the dormant embryos and rouses them to activity. They begin to wiggle about in their eggs, and their motion causes the egg mass to break

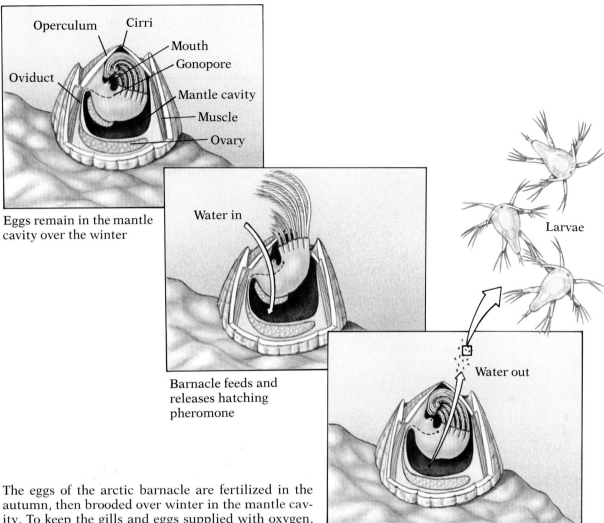

Eggs remain in the mantle cavity over the winter

Operculum   Cirri
Mouth
Gonopore
Oviduct
Mantle cavity
Muscle
Ovary

Water in

Barnacle feeds and releases hatching pheromone

Water out

Larvae

Eggs hatch and larvae leave the cavity

The eggs of the arctic barnacle are fertilized in the autumn, then brooded over winter in the mantle cavity. To keep the gills and eggs supplied with oxygen, the barnacle pumps water in and out of its mantle cavity by swinging its body upward and backward, then downward and forward, while raising and lowering the operculum, the hard plate over the top of the body. During feeding, it extends and withdraws its six pairs of limbs, or cirri, in rhythm with the pumping cycle; they act as a net that captures planktonic organisms. After the eggs hatch in response to the hatching pheromone, they are able to leave the mantle cavity when the downward swing of the barnacle body displaces water from the cavity.

down. The eggs hatch and release the larvae into the cavity. From here they can swim out into the sea and away from their sessile (immobile) mother.

There is considerable evidence that this barnacle's hatching pheromone is a prostaglandin. Prostaglandins are a group of closely related compounds found in both invertebrates and vertebrates. In man and other mammals the prostaglandins are extremely important owing to their diverse physiological effects. They excite smooth muscle, depress blood pressure, and play a critical role in metabolism, in reproduction, and in production of inflammation. These observations in *B. balanoides* are the first indication of a function for prostaglandins in invertebrates.

A Signal to Settle

The larval *Balanus balanoides* start out as free-swimming creatures, but later they settle down, attach themselves to a surface, and develop into adults. At the time of settling there is a second chemical signal that influences where they establish themselves. It is difficult to get these barnacles to colonize a fresh surface, because the larvae tend to select a site where other barnacles have already settled. This behavior results from an attractant pheromone. Barnacles and other arthropods have in their hard outer covering, or cuticle, a group of related proteins, called arthropodins, that slowly leach into the surrounding water. The larvae of *B. balanoides* are attracted to these arthropodins and tend to settle on a surface from which they come.

The arthropodins from various arthropods are chemically similar in structure, but not identical. Closely related proteins from different species often have structures with very similar sequences of amino acids, but with the occasional replacement of a particular amino acid by a different one. The barnacle larvae are most strongly attracted by the protein of their own species, but they will also respond to the protein from other arthropods.

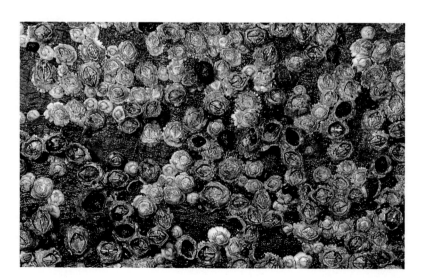

Adult arctic barnacles on a rock face with many smaller young barnacles that have settled more recently.

A Hatching Pheromone: Embryos Signal Their Mother

Another crustacean that uses a pheromone to control egg hatching is *Rhitropanopeus harrisii,* a crab native to estuaries that are common along the very irregular coast of North Carolina. In *B. balanoides* the hatching pheromone passed from female to embryo, but in *R. harrisii* it moves in the opposite direction. The embryos themselves provide the signal that controls the hatching of their own eggs. We owe our knowledge of this strange system to the efforts of Richard B. Forward, Jr., and his coworkers at Duke University, who have studied crustaceans along the North Carolina coast for many years.

As do other crabs, the female of this species lays fertilized eggs, attaches them to the lower surface of her abdomen, and carries them about until they hatch. It is common for the hatching of crab eggs to be coordinated with tidal, light–dark, or lunar cycles, and to be synchronized so that a female releases all her larvae over a short period. In *R. harrisii* the light–dark cycle is controlling, and the eggs hatch in the hours just after dark. The process begins with the female crab performing a repeated and distinctive stereotyped action. She stands up on her walking legs and flexes her abdomen back and forth in a pumping action. This physically breaks unhatched eggs and brings about nearly simultaneous release of all the larvae.

Experiments with water in which eggs had recently hatched, but which was free of both eggs and larvae, revealed that the "pumping response" of the female is triggered by a pheromone present in this water. Chemical analysis of the water and careful research revealed the origin and action of this signal from eggs to mother. As the time for hatching approaches, small peptides accumulate in the eggs. These peptides probably come from stepwise breakdown of proteins in the membranes of the maturing egg mass. At hatching time the eggs become fragile, and normal movements of the female or embryos break a few of them. These ruptured eggs release both their larvae and the newly formed small peptides into the water. Certain of the peptides then act as a pheromone to elicit the pumping response from the female.

The female's energetic physical action brings about the rupture of the main body of

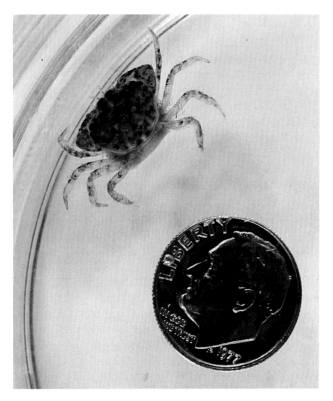

An adult estuarine crab *Rhitropanopeus harrisii* next to a dime (the diameter of which is 18 millimeters).

eggs and the release of their larvae. As more eggs break, the concentration of the pheromone in the water increases, and the female responds to the stronger signal by pumping more vigorously. While a female carrying immature eggs will give the pumping response to the pheromone, this does not rupture her eggs before their time. For the eggs to hatch, not only must the female perform the pumping action, but the egg shells must already be weakened and the egg mass broken down. All these changes take place as the eggs complete their development, with the consequence that natural hatching is accomplished quickly once the eggs are mature and a few begin to open.

Forward and his co-workers had isolated the active material from water in which eggs had hatched and found that it contained a mixture of dipeptides and tripeptides, which they wished to identify. Because it is easier to identify small amounts of amino acids than peptides, Forward converted the mixture of peptides chemically into its constituent amino acids. On analysis he found eight different amino acids. The problem now was to decide how these eight amino acids had been joined into peptides and which of these peptides functioned as the pumping signal. Many small peptides are commercially available, and it was convenient to solve the problem by trial and error. Forward tested the response of female crabs carrying eggs to eleven di- and tripeptides that could be formed from the isolated amino acids; he also tested two peptides containing a ninth amino acid that had not been found. Several peptides, and also several amino acids, showed measurable activity in eliciting the pumping response, but only one compound was highly active. This was the dipeptide leucylarginine, which had a response threshold of 43 picograms per milliliter. By comparing the structures of leucylarginine and the other less active peptides, Forward was

$$H_3C\!\!\diagdown\atop{H_3C}\!\!\diagup CHCH_2\underset{NH_2}{CH}\overset{O}{\overset{\|}{C}}NHCHCOOH\atop{CH_2CH_2CH_2NH\underset{\|}{C}NH_2}$$

$$NH$$

Leucylarginine

able to gain some information about the size and shape of the receptor in the mother crab that interacts with the pheromone.

Eliciting the Experience of a Lifetime

There is another crab in which a sex pheromone of unknown chemical structure induces striking courtship behavior in the male. *Callinectes sapidus* is the common blue crab of commerce. It is sold as a foodstuff, either as the "hard-shell crab" or, just after molting, as the "soft-shell crab." Its reproductive behavior is under the control of a pheromone that appears in the urine of the female just before she matures. The male detects the pheromone with sense organs located on his first antennae (crabs have two pairs of antennae), and he responds to its signal with an odd courtship display. He spreads his claws apart in front, he extends his walking legs, and in the rear he raises his swimming legs and waves them from side to side over the top of his shell. Having attracted the female's attention with this antic performance, he then grabs her, tucks her under his body, and carries her around wherever he goes for several days. Soon she undergoes her maturity molt, and immediately afterward copulation takes place. The male continues to tote the female about for several more days. In the normal course of events, this is the single mating experience in

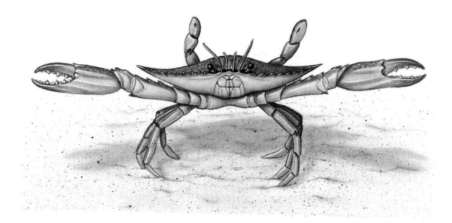

The courtship display of the male blue crab.

the life of a female blue crab. Despite considerable effort, investigators have not yet succeeded in isolating and identifying the active pheromone in female urine that sets off these spectacular events.

Alarms That Scatter

Like crustaceans, arachnids are a class of the arthropods; they include spiders, scorpions, ticks, and mites. To many people these are rather repugnant beasts, and over the centuries many human cultures have viewed scorpions as a particular abomination. Perhaps this negative attitude has contributed to our relative ignorance of the use of chemical signals in arachnids. Chemical communication seems to play an important role in the mating of scorpions, but nothing is yet known in detail, and until fairly recently it was thought that spiders made no use of pheromones at all. This seemed believable, because spiders have developed complex systems of tactile communication, exploiting vibrations of their silken webs and draglines to convey messages of many

sorts. However, evidence of a role for pheromones is now appearing, at least in some kinds of spiders. Both airborne chemicals and pheromones applied to silk seem to be employed, mostly by the female to attract the male. Little more is known at present.

In contrast, ticks and mites make extensive use of chemical communication, and the body of behavioral and chemical information here is beginning to grow. Ticks are larger than mites; in both, the adults have eight walking legs, simple eyes, and no antennae. These are characteristics that they share with spiders and that distinguish them from insects. They are typically parasitic organisms, and mites, like nematodes, have parasitized almost every species of plant and animal larger than themselves. One mite about half a millimeter (0.02 inch) long makes its home in hair follicles of the human face. Another inhabits the respiratory system of honey bees. More than 20,000 species of mites have been described, but this is assumed to be too small a fraction of the whole to permit any reliable estimate of the total number of species extant.

Because they are parasites, ticks and mites, again like nematodes, are an economi-

These respiratory tubules inside a honey
bee are infested with the mite *Acarapis
woodi*, which is a serious problem for
beekeepers in some parts of the world.

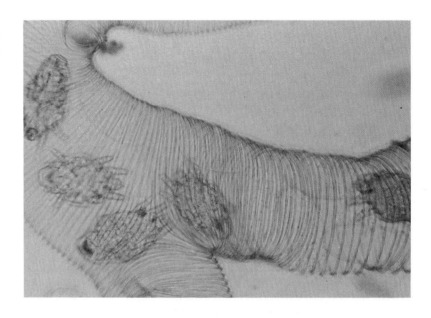

cally important group. They destroy stored
products such as grain, they infest fruit and
many other foodstuffs, and they carry several
human and animal diseases, such as Rocky
Mountain spotted fever, Lyme disease, tulare-
mia, and Texas cattle fever. A mite is also
responsible for scabies, a human disease char-
acterized by a skin irritation accompanied by
a maddening itch. It was rightly linked with
the mite *Sarcoptes scabiei* in seventeenth-
century Italy and thus became the first human
disease with a recognized cause. The notoriety
of ticks and mites has encouraged active study
of their biology and examination of the role of
chemical communication in their lives. The
pheromones that have received most attention
cause aggregation, signal alarm, or control
aspects of reproduction.

Some of the pheromones employed by
ticks and mites are not species-specific. Furthermore, they present a situation reminiscent
of the widely distributed hydrocarbons that
are the sex attractants of brown algae. The
same compounds are made by several related
species but do not function as pheromones in
all of them. These substances are released
when the mites sense danger, causing other
mites to flee the area. Note that alarm pheromones may bear one of two different sorts of
messages. Some, including the present example, provoke a rapid evacuation of an area,
just as a fire alarm does. Others serve to alert
and rally those who receive the message.
These signals raise an alarm that brings individuals together to mount an attack. (Ants and
bees have pheromones of this latter sort, and
we will discuss them later.)

Several mites make a compound known as
2-hydroxy-6-methylbenzaldehyde, but it is active as an alarm pheromone only in *Tyro-
phagus perniciosus*, a familiar greenhouse pest
that infests members of the gourd family. A
related greenhouse mite, *T. neiswanderi*, uses
a blend of long-chain hydrocarbons containing
a double bond as an alarm pheromone. A similar mixture also appears in the cheese mite,

T. putrescentiae, but here it is without pheromonal activity. However, in the cheese mite and several other species, neryl formate serves as an alarm pheromone. Finally, in *T. similis* the alarm pheronome is isopiperitenone, a compound previously familiar to chemists as a constituent of an aromatic plant oil. These facts seem confusing. Several kinds of compounds act as alarm pheromones in these mites, and we know too little to see any pattern here. We need a great deal more information before making useful generalizations about these signals.

Signals That Gather

The opposite kind of message is broadcast by certain pheromones of many species of ticks. This message is: Assemble now! These ticks spend much of their time as blood-sucking parasites on various mammals or birds. The pheromone is deposited on the natural substrate of the tick off its host, that is, on bushes or on the ground or wherever the tick lives when it has no host. This pheromone arrests wandering ticks on contact, causing them to aggregate in tight clusters and remain quiescent. Presumably, such behavior protects the ticks during stressful periods of living without a host and improves their chances of surviving until they can find a new host and resume a parasitic existence. Here again, a single compound is active in a number of species. To accommodate this aggregating function, the pheromone ideally should be a nonvolatile compound that persists on the substrate and in the environment. Guanine, a nitrogen-containing compound that has these properties, is the common assembly pheromone for a variety of ticks.

A remarkable characteristic of this aggregating response of ticks is that it is dependent upon the local humidity. This surprising fact was discovered by investigators at the International Centre of Insect Physiology and Ecology in Nairobi, Kenya. During a rainy period these scientists found that they could not reproduce their earlier results on the aggregation of the fowl tick *Argas* in response to guanine. They then undertook controlled experiments and discovered an unusual relationship between humidity and the response to the pheromone. At low humidity *Argas* responds to guanine by aggregating, but at high humidity the effect is reversed and guanine stimulates dispersion.

This change with humidity perhaps serves to solve a problem that is inherent in use of a stable, persistent compound, such as guanine, to promote aggregation: How is the message turned off when it is no longer advantageous for the ticks to aggregate? It may be that periods of low humidity and accompanying high temperature are particularly stressful for the ticks, and that aggregation minimizes water loss in ticks massed under these conditions. When the weather changes and the humidity is higher, there may be less advantage to the ticks in remaining in a quiescent group. If the benefits of aggregation are in fact dependent on the weather in this fashion, the novel change in response with humidity is obviously advantageous. With improved weather, the ticks are free to wander and search out a host.

The Nairobi scientists have noted three possible mechanisms to account for the change of message with humidity. First, there could be a chemical change in guanine at high humidity, so that it is transformed into a different substance with a different message. Second, the tick could combine information received from its pheromone receptors with that from putative humidity receptors to yield a final message that depends on integration of these two signals. Third, the receptor protein in the tick could undergo a change at high humidity, so that its interaction with guanine yields an altered signal. The first possibility is easily tested, and in fact guanine suffers no chemical change as a function of humidity. A choice between the other two possibilities, or some alternative mechanism, is an open problem for future research.

For a number of years sex attractant pheromones were known from ticks but not from mites. A compound known as β-acaridial is now recognized as an attractant for *Caloglyphus polyphyllae*, a mite that lives in stored products. Investigators at the University of Tsukuba in Japan have carried out extensive studies on a variety of mite pheromones, and they isolated this compound while searching for an alarm pheromone in *C. polyphyllae*. They tested their newly found substance for alarm activity in an appropriate, simple bioassay. They placed a small drop of test solution on a piece of filter paper where both sexes of *Caloglyphus* were feeding. A positive alarm response would have sent the mites scurrying away from the droplet and to the edges of the paper. Instead, as the solution wet the paper, male mites stopped feeding, became visibly agitated, and began racing across the paper toward the pheromone, copulating with any females they encountered on the way. Far from an alarm signal, β-acaridial is a potent sex attractant.

β-Acaridial and a closely related compound also produced by mites, α-acaridial, are also antifungal agents that kill several common fungi, including *Penicillium vermiculatum*, *Aspergilis niger*, and *Fusarium oxysporum*. This is an intriguing property, because these mites live in and feed on stored products such as wheat and other grains and they share their habitats with fungi that compete with them for the same food. The acaridials must provide the mites the additional benefit of reducing the populations of these undesirable fungi.

A Hierarchy of Mating Signals

The widely distributed American dog tick *Dermacentor variabilis* is probably the tick most likely to be encountered in everyday life in the United States. On a visit to the woods either man or dog can pick up several specimens. The dog tick can be more than a minor nuisance, because it transmits Rocky Mountain spotted fever. This readily available tick has been the object of extensive scrutiny, and largely through the continuing investigations of Daniel E. Sonenshine and his co-workers at Old Dominion University in Virginia, we are now familiar with three different pheromones that direct the ticks' reproductive behavior. These signals control a hierarchy of mating responses.

The first of these three reproductive pheromones is a potent attractant released by the female. The active compound in *D. variabilis*, as well as in many other species, is 2,6-dichlorophenol. Related compounds are the sex attractants of still other ticks. Dichlorophenol, which is a common laboratory chemical, is secreted in oily solution onto the outer surface of the female tick, and from there it slowly evaporates into the atmosphere. Not only does this attractant lack species specificity, but in some species both male and female ticks are about equally attracted to it. This use of a single compound as a sex attractant in many related species raises the prospect of confusion over who is attracted to whom.

The same problem appears in insects, where it has been examined in some detail. When insect species share both an attractant and the same range, there is often some difference in their rhythm of production of the pheromone and responsiveness to it. When one species is making use of the signal, the other species is in the wrong phase of its life cycle or otherwise not interested. By preventing the

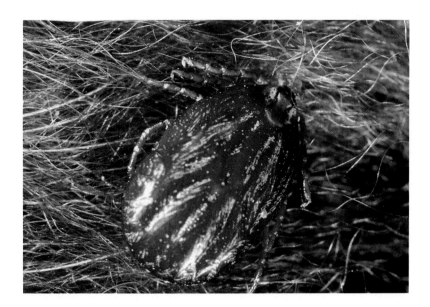

The common American dog tick *Dermacentor variabilis*. This species thrives over a large portion of North America.

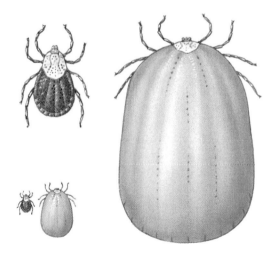

The common dog tick before and after a blood meal. The smaller pictures indicate the actual size of the tick.

two species from mating, this arrangement helps maintain their separate identity. In contrast to this effective segregation typically enjoyed by insects, interspecific mating does take place among some species of ticks that share a sex attractant in the same living space. As we shall see, *D. variabilis* has another mechanism to discourage interspecific mating.

D. variabilis begins reproductive activity only after male and female have found a suitable host and started to feed. Dichlorophenol then spreads through the environment from the female and summons the male tick. On making contact with her, the male encounters the second pheromone. This is an oily compound on her body surface. It prompts the male to mount the female and initiate exploratory behavior.

For *D. variabilis* the active mounting pheromone is cholesteryl oleate. This is the ester formed between oleic acid and cholesterol, a

Cholesteryl oleate, the mounting pheromone of the dog tick, is a long oleic acid chain (green) joined to cholesterol (tan).

steroid that we encountered earlier. Oleic acid is one of the common fatty acids, long-chain compounds with a carboxyl group at one end, that are found in dietary fats. Cholesteryl oleate is one of the forms in which cholesterol regularly circulates in mammalian blood systems. The ticks pick up this fatty substance in their diet of mammalian blood, so this is an example of a pheromone that the organism ingests rather than synthesizes. We will have more to say about such situations later. The cholesteryl oleate molecule is sufficiently large to be quite nonvolatile, and consequently this substance does not evaporate and diffuse through the environment but remains on the female tick. For this reason the male makes contact with it only after reaching the female. Cholesterol itself is a crystalline compound that melts only at the high temperature of 150°C. Owing to the long oleic acid chain, cholesteryl oleate is a fatty substance that melts to a heavy oil at 44°C, just a few degrees above mammalian body temperature. It should form a greasy coating on the female tick.

The presence of cholesteryl oleate on the female had been known for some time before the compound was recognized as having a crit-

ical biological function. It had been identified spectroscopically but was long regarded as merely a waste product. Because the feeding female tick takes in quantities of cholesteryl oleate with her blood meal, scientists assumed that she simply excreted the compound and that it collected on her body surface without serving any purpose there.

We now know that cholesteryl oleate signals the feeding female's readiness to mate and stimulates the male to mount her. This means that host availability and successful parasitism are prerequisites for reproduction. It seems probable that originally cholesteryl oleate was indeed merely a waste product of the feeding tick, and that subsequent evolution converted it into an important reproductive signal. About one-tenth of the amount of cholesteryl oleate typically found on the surface of a feeding female will induce the male to mount. In general, there are many situations in which organisms secrete or excrete substances in connection with some specific physiological state or activity, and the concept that such compounds could evolve into signals to other members of the community is an attractive one.

The mounting pheromone prompts the male tick to move about over the body of the female. In this exploration he probes her genital opening or gonopore. Here he comes upon the copulatory pheromone, and only on detecting this third signal does he initiate copulation. This pheromone is a mixture of compounds that are synthesized in the female reproductive tract and then move onto the external genital surface where the male discovers them during his exploratory activities.

This biological setting, along with the copulatory response, dictated a relatively laborious bioassay for identification of the active compounds in the copulatory pheromone. For the bioassay to work, the male tick had to encounter the test substances under circumstances appropriate for his natural response. This meant making use of female ticks, and for the bioassay to be meaningful, these females had to be totally free of their copulatory pheromones.

To get females free of pheromone, Sonenshine and his research group surgically neutered female ticks by severing the vagina from the gonopore and then completely removing the vagina and uterus. Without these organs, the females could no longer synthesize the copulatory signal. After surgery, the investigators painstakingly removed all residual traces of copulatory pheromone from the bodies of the ticks by first washing the gonopore with organic solvent and then scraping the surface clean. To demonstrate that this entire procedure had been successful, they released a sexually active male near each neutered female after letting the female attach to and feed on a rabbit. Because she had fed on blood, the neutered female was coated with mounting pheromone, which stimulated the male's exploratory activity. If he copulated with the female, she was discarded. The male was permitted three separate opportunities with the female, and each neutered female was tested against five different males.

The Sonenshine group then used the female ticks that survived this stringent test in the bioassay. The investigators applied a standardized amount of solution or extract to be assayed to the gonopore of the neutered female and allowed the tick to reattach to its rabbit host. Twenty-four hours later they placed a sexually active male next to the female. If he copulated with her, they scored a positive result. Again, they gave each male three opportunities with the female carrying the test substance and employed five different males in each bioassay. The combined 15 results gave a final score for each female used in the test. After the bioassay, they dissected each neutered female to verify that the gonopore was intact and that the vagina and uterus had indeed been successfully removed in the initial surgical operation.

This intricate bioassay revealed that the most active components of the natural pheromone were fatty acids with 14, 16, 18, and 20 carbon atoms. Synthetic mixtures of these acids produce the copulatory response, but the natural signal probably also contains additional components that have not yet been identified. Because neither the attractant pheromone, dichlorophenol, nor the mounting pheromone, cholesteryl oleate, is species-specific, male dog ticks will approach and mount females of other species that employ these same signals. Normally, however, they copulate only with females of their own species, presumably because they do not find the necessary copulatory pheromone in other species. This third signal provides the special mechanism that discourages these ticks from mating with other species.

In at least one instance, however, there is some other mechanism to prevent interspecific mating by dog ticks, but it is not yet certain just how this operates. *D. variabilis* lives together in nature with a closely related tick, *Dermacentor andersoni*. These ticks rarely mate with one another, and no one has identified hybrids of the two species. For both species, dichlorophenol is the natural attractant and cholesteryl oleate is the mounting pheromone. With this in mind, we would not expect the two species to use the same copulatory pheromone.

Sonenshine and his students used their neutered-female bioassay separately with each species to identify its copulatory pheromone. Although the investigators found minor differences in composition of the pheromone, they discovered that the two ticks produce pheromones containing very similar mixtures of fatty acids and that they respond to the same compounds. The one striking difference between the two is that *D. variabilis* yielded an average of 25 nanograms of copulatory pheromone per female, while the amount from *D. andersoni* was 297 nanograms. This twelvefold difference suggests that perhaps *D. variabilis* is more sensitive to the pheromone, and that this difference in sensitivity provides the basis for species discrimination in these two ticks.

In general, it is not unusual for an excessively high level of a pheromone to produce an effect unlike the natural concentration. We saw a case of this in the paralysis of the nematode *H. glycines* induced by unnaturally high concentrations of vanillic acid. It may be that for *D. variabilis* males, the high concentration of the pheromone produced by *D. andersoni* females is repugnant, and that *D. andersoni* males cannot detect the lower level of the pheromone available in *D. variabilis* females.

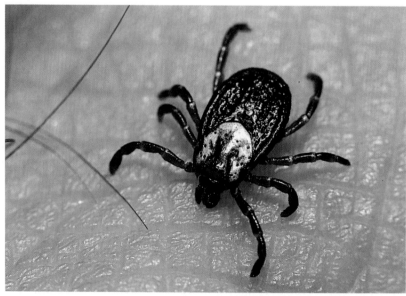

A female wood tick *Dermacentor andersoni*. This species lives in western North America, and like its relative the dog tick it carries Rocky Mountain spotted fever.

Alternatively, some yet unidentified components of the copulatory pheromone may distinguish the two signals. In some way the two species of ticks keep themselves apart.

Behaviorists are accumulating evidence for pheromones in many other invertebrates, and chemists have structural information on a few of the pheromones employed by these organisms. Unquestionably, in the years ahead new investigations will turn up whole systems of invertebrate pheromones analogous to the signals of the dog tick. It is time now, however, for us to focus attention on the insects, the single class of arthropods that accounts for most of the known invertebrates and for most of what we know about pheromones.

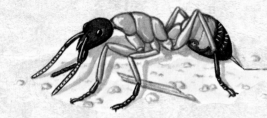

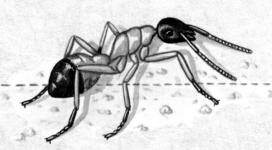

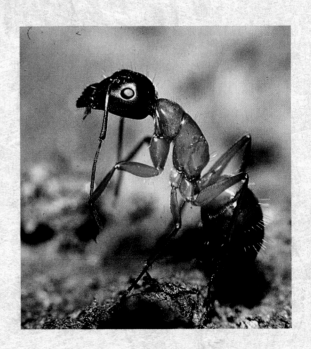

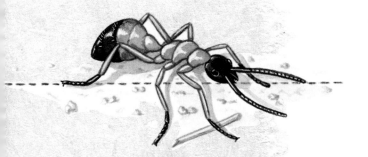

4

COOPERATION AND DECEPTION AMONG THE INSECTS

*M*ost of what we know about pheromones comes from studies of chemical communication in insects. Scientists studying pheromones in these creatures need not worry about running out of new material, as insects make up a whole world all by themselves. Experts offer widely differing numbers, but there are at least 800,000 *described* species of insects. Recent extrapolations from studies of tropical rain forests suggest that there may be as many as thirty million species of insects! Beetles alone make up about a quarter of all known animals, and the insects as a whole account for some 70 percent of the de-scribed species. There are about 10^{18} individual insects in the world. With a global population of five thousand million humans, that is two hundred million insects for each person on earth.

Insects provide some of mankind's worst natural enemies and also contribute a few very close friends. Agricultural damage from natural predators, which are chiefly insects, amounts overall to about 13 percent of the potential crop. In particular instances the loss can be much greater. An infestation of Colorado potato beetles *(Leptinotarsa decemlineata)* early in the growing season can totally destroy a potato crop. The number and variety of agricultural pests is impressive; worldwide, cotton is subject to assault by more than 1,300 species of insects. The cost in lost crops is huge, and the direct cost of the endless combat against these predators is enormous. There is also an indirect cost connected with this problem and our human response to it. The price of the social and environmental damage attributable to the use of insecticides, damage such as water pollution, pesticide residues in food, and the endangerment of nontargeted species, including man, is estimated to amount to more than eight hundred million dollars annually in the United States alone. This environmental cost receives increasing public and scientific attention, but the worldwide peril it represents is still widely underestimated.

The other group of prominent insect enemies are the carriers of human and animal diseases. These insects transmit the viruses, bacteria, and other agents that cause several serious disorders, and typically the insect is a necessary link in spreading these diseases. The best-known of these is probably malaria, which is caused by parasites carried by certain kinds of mosquitoes. Also included among insect-carried diseases are bubonic plague, yellow fever, typhus, anthrax, African sleeping sickness, and several other horrors.

To balance these insect-borne miseries we should recall that mankind has a long-standing and highly beneficial relationship with the silkworm moth *Bombyx mori* and the honey bee *Apis mellifera*. There are records of bee-keeping from the Old Kingdom of ancient Egypt (roughly 2500 B.C.), and cave paintings depict humans robbing honey from the hives of wild bees thousands of years earlier. Tradition places the origin of silk in China also at about 2500 B.C., but there is physical evidence from neolithic archaeological sites suggesting that silkworms were being cultivated much earlier. By the ninth century B.C., silk was sufficiently widely known and valued in China to be in use as a medium of exchange.

In addition to these two species that have achieved worldwide economic and cultural importance, there are instances of insects beneficial to humankind on a more local and humble scale. There is, for example, the vidalia beetle *Rodolia cardinalis*, brought to California in 1889 in one of the earliest and most successful efforts at biological pest control. This beetle was introduced into California citrus groves to combat another insect, cottonycushion scale *(Icerya purchasi)*, which now after one hundred years is still under control, thanks to the vidalia beetle's prodigious and specialized appetite for the pest.

Many monographs and articles about pheromones deal only with chemical signals in insects. The study of chemical communication focuses on insects in part because agricultural pests are so important economically. The desirability of restraining insect predation is clear, as is the cost of the continued heavy use of insecticides. In these circumstances researchers are attracted to the possibility of controlling pests by deploying natural chemical signals. In principle relatively small

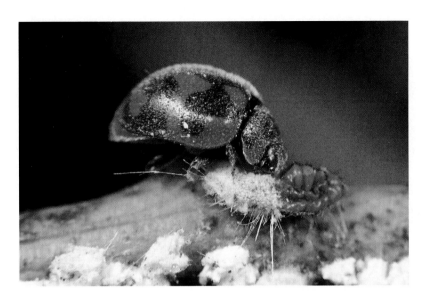

An adult vidalia beetle feeding on cottonycushion scale, its favorite food.

amounts of generally nontoxic substances could control insect pests without destroying other organisms. These considerations have provided funds, interest, and motivation for thorough studies of pheromonal systems in insect pests for the past thirty years. A large portion of these pests are larval butterflies or moths—vast armies of caterpillars with insatiable appetites. The desire to control these larvae has led to more than 1,200 research papers on pheromones in Lepidoptera over the past twenty-five years. The widespread pheromonal control of agricultural pests is not yet a reality, although there are specific instances of encouraging practical success.

Insect pheromones are convenient for chemical studies in other ways. In general the compounds employed as signals by insects are chemically simple, and thus it has been relatively easy to determine their structures and then synthesize them. The development of gas chromatography starting in the mid-1950s provided an excellent tool for analyzing and purifying these compounds just at the time that interest was rising in the area. This technique is particularly suited for handling the relatively volatile, thermally stable compounds that usually serve as insect pheromones. An important refinement was the coupling of gas chromatography with mass spectrometry. Not only can nanogram amounts of material give useful spectra with a minimum of manipulation, but computers can now be used to compare the results with libraries of the previously determined spectra of thousands of compounds. For the simple compounds found in many insect pheromones, these procedures can often lead to quick and secure identification.

By the early 1980s 731 insect species had been examined and had yielded 323 different compounds used as chemical signals. We have a more completely integrated picture of chemical signaling here than we have in other organisms. We know about the structure of the glands that produce the pheromones, the re-

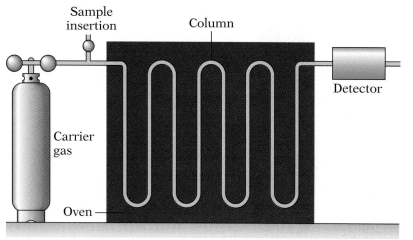

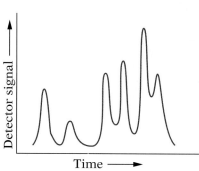

Gas chromatography is a technique for separating, identifying, and measuring the quantity of each volatile component of a mixture. A sample of the mixture is injected by a valve into a long capillary column, through which is passed an inert carrier gas, in most cases helium. The walls of the capillary column are lined with a thin layer of a silicone oil in which the different components have different solubility. The rate of passage of each component through the column depends on its solubility in the silicone oil, so that each component travels at a specific rate and emerges from the column at a specific time. The output stream passes through a detector that generates a signal for each component. The size of the signal corresponds to the amount of the component present.

ceptors that detect them, and the pathways from detection to behavior. There is information on just how some attractant pheromones stimulate an insect to fly toward the signal source. For certain groups of insects links are apparent between evolutionary relationships and the chemical composition of pheromones. There are data on the specificity of pheromones in closely related species and how this specificity helps these species maintain separate identities. We have learned how an enzyme in the olfactory apparatus destroys a pheromone after it has been detected. Investi-

gators have identified genes that control the synthesis of specific pheromones and have studied them in depth. For investigators working in another direction, enough is known about signals in certain groups of insects to apply information theory and correlate the complexity of a pheromone molecule with its information content and the specificity of a signal. With insects we are beginning to fit chemical communication into the broader themes of biology.

Here we can only sample this mass of data, choosing a few topics to illustrate how chemical communication works in insects and what we know about it. An obvious place to start is with the first pheromone to be identified chemically, because this achievement had an enormous effect on the subsequent maturation of this area of science. It is worthwhile to consider this work in some detail, particularly because it was carried out before the development of modern spectroscopic and analytical techniques.

Bombykol, the Silkworm Moth's Attractant

By the late 1930s it was clear that chemicals can mediate communication between members of a species. The German organic chemist Adolph Butenandt became interested in the possibility of isolating and identifying such a compound, although it was certain that the technical difficulties in the undertaking would be formidable. Adolph Butenandt had been

one of the pioneers in isolating and determining the structures of the steroidal sex hormones, and he shared in the Nobel Prize for Chemistry in 1939 at the age of 36. Other chemists had shown little interest in identifying a chemical signal, and it is a measure of Butenandt's intellectual breadth that he moved in this unexplored direction.

Butenandt chose to investigate the silkworm moth *Bombyx mori* and its attractant pheromone, which came to be known as bombykol. This was a fortunate marriage of scientist and problem. More than twenty years would pass before the structure of bombykol was learned, and without Butenandt's reputation and ability it could have taken even longer. Few investigators could have sustained their effort or elicited financial support so long for an investigation with so few positive results along the way. In addition to the problem of funding, the disruptions of the Second World War, and the logistical problems in obtaining the large numbers of silkworm moths needed, Butenandt faced biological problems

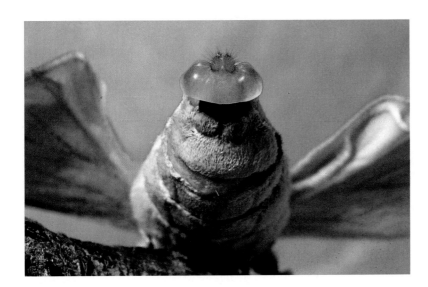

The female silkworm moth releases bombykol from a pair of scent sacs located at the tip of her abdomen.

in devising an appropriate bioassay, and chemical problems in working with what was, at the time, a very small amount of material.

The silkworm moth, with its attractant bombykol, was a convenient choice for Butenandt and his coworkers. Silkworms were already grown on a large scale for the commercial production of silk, and raising silkworms was a popular hobby in Europe at the time. The attractant is contained in a pair of glands at the tip of the abdomen of the female, and for the early investigations several thousand glands sufficed to provide the active material on which to begin fractionation. At the time, enough insects could be bought each year in northern Germany from silkworm hobbyists. As the research progressed, more and more females were needed, and Butenandt began to turn to commercial silkworm growers for larger supplies. Unfortunately, as the demand for silkworms rose in the laboratory, the supply dwindled in the market. The German climate is relatively unfavorable for large-scale culture of *Bombyx*, and the postwar development of artificial fibers had effectively destroyed the German silk industry by about 1952. Eventually, Butenandt located stable sources of silkworms in Italy and Japan.

After some seventeen years of study, the final isolation effort began in 1956 with more than a million silk cocoons, enough to yield about 90 kilograms (200 pounds) of silk. These cocoons furnished 500,000 female moths. This vast number of moths was necessary to supply enough bombykol for rigorous elucidation of its chemical structure. The minimum amount of a totally novel compound necessary for identification by the techniques of the day was a few milligrams. Much more might be needed if the structure was complex. After painstaking, extensive fractionation, the glands from the 500,000 females yielded 6.4 milligrams of bombykol.

The bioassay guiding this purification work depended on the behavior of the male moth. Although he cannot fly and ordinarily remains quiescent when isolated, the male beats his wings in a "flutter dance" when exposed to the pheromone. The German chemists used this behavior in a semiquantitative bioassay by testing solutions of the material in question on groups of 30 to 60 males. The particular fraction to be assayed was presented in a dilution series of test solutions, with each successive solution one-tenth the concentration of the previous one. The particular concentration of a tested fraction that elicited the flutter dance in about 50 percent of the group of males was defined as containing the "sex pheromone unit" (SPU), expressed in micrograms of material contained in one milliliter, or $\mu g/ml$, of test solution.

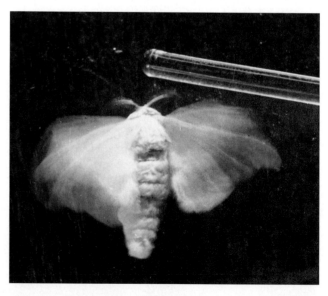

A male silkworm moth flutters his wings rapidly in response to a minute amount of bombykol on the glass rod.

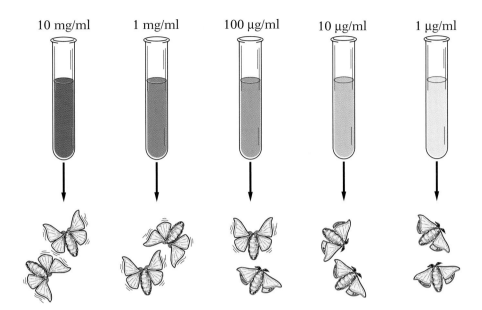

10 mg/ml   1 mg/ml   100 µg/ml   10 µg/ml   1 µg/ml

The bioassay used in purifying bombykol depended on the response of male moths to a series of test samples that differed tenfold in concentration. In this illustration half the moths are responding at a concentration of 100 micrograms of sample per milliliter of solution, giving an SPU of 100 µg/ml.

As the fractionation steps removed extraneous, inactive matter, and the active pheromone became purer, the weight necessary to produce the flutter dance decreased, and with it the SPU decreased. For example, the first step in the purification of bombykol gave 125 grams (g) of crude material with an SPU of 100 µg/ml. Two more purification steps reduced the total weight to 7.3 g with an SPU of 1×10^{-4} µg/ml (100 picograms per milliliter). While the total weight decreased seventeenfold, the SPU went down (improved) by a factor of one million. The rapid decrease of the SPU indicated the effectiveness of the purification scheme by showing that inactive material was selectively being removed. That is, purification was taking place! Chemically pure bombykol ultimately proved to have an SPU of 1×10^{-12} µg/ml (one millionth of a picogram per milliliter).

In the bioassay the chemists used a group of males, rather than only one, to average individual variation in response among moths.

Defining the SPU as the response by 50 percent of the males takes further account of these individual differences and also helps provide a roughly linear relationship between the observed response and the amount of material producing it. This sounds similar in principle to bioassays that we have met earlier, and in fact the techniques used in assaying bombykol became commonplace in subsequent studies. In the early days of the silkworm work, however, these ideas and methods were new. Later efforts took advantage of this pioneering research.

The more sensitive the bioassay, the more information it provides to guide the fractionation. Butenandt and his coworkers looked into two improvements designed to enhance sensitivity in their bioassay. One was to test only those males that responded exuberantly to the pheromone. This simple change proved particularly beneficial in later stages of the isolation. The other modification was to incorporate electrophysiological techniques into the bioassay. Instead of employing whole male moths, the German scientists could use antennae freshly excised from males. By inserting two steel or glass microelectrodes into an isolated antenna, the scientists could record nerve impulses from receptor cells of the antenna. These recordings became known as "electroantennograms." When antennae with attached electrodes were exposed to bombykol fractions, there was an increase in the amplitude and frequency of nerve impulses from the receptor cells. This procedure showed promise, but it was not refined for routine application in the isolation of bombykol. It later became a standard technique in analysis of insect pheromones, particularly owing to the efforts of Wendell L. Roelofs of the New York State Agricultural Experiment Station at Geneva, New York.

Following the guidance of their bioassay, the German scientists were able to prepare a fraction of natural material with high pheromonal activity. This fraction contained only one active component. The next step was to convert this fraction into the pure active compound. With the equipment and techniques available today, bombykol would be purified by gas chromatography, and its structure could probably be determined spectroscopically in short order. These tools were not in routine use in the 1950s, and Butenandt had to purify bombykol using chemical techniques and then determine its structure by a combination of chemical reactions, the limited spectroscopic methods available, and independent synthesis.

The small amount of pheromone available made identifying bombykol a demanding task, but finally it became clear what its structure must be. Butenandt's research group independently synthesized bombykol, along with the three closely related compounds having other arrangements of the carbon chains about the double bonds. Butenandt and his collaborators

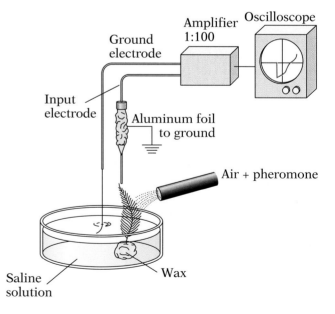

The electroantennogram depends on the high sensitivity of the male moth antennae to the female sex pheromone. Clean filtered air blows continuously over the antenna at a constant rate; into this air stream, the investigator introduces test samples. The antenna responds to the pheromone with an immediate electrical signal, which is amplified and displayed on an oscilloscope. This antennogram set-up can be used as a rapid, routine detector for fractions coming directly from a gas chromatograph.

$$CH_3CH_2CH_2 \overset{H}{\underset{H}{C}} = \overset{H}{\underset{}{C}} \quad \overset{H}{\underset{}{C}} = \overset{}{\underset{H}{C}} \quad CH_2CH_2CH_2CH_2CH_2CH_2CH_2CH_2CH_2OH$$

Bombykol

What does it take to make a moth flutter? The three compounds with other arrangements about the double bonds made moths flutter in the bioassay, but only at concentrations between a thousand million and ten million million times greater than that of bombykol. The bombykol receptor can detect the differences these changes make in molecular shape.

tested all four of these compounds in the flutter-dance bioassay. Each compound provoked a response, but only bombykol made the male moths flutter at the infinitesimal concentration available in the natural world.

Biological Investigations with Bombykol

Knowledge of the chemical structure of bombykol encouraged experimental approaches to several new questions. How does the female synthesize and control production of bombykol? That is, what are the biochemical steps in converting molecules available from her diet into bombykol, and what factors control operation of these steps? What triggers the female's release of bombykol? There are also questions about what happens when the male moth receives the pheromone. How does the male antenna recognize bombykol? What does the pheromone do that causes the male to fly to the female?

Investigators formulated experiments to answer many of these questions more easily

once the structure of the pheromone was known and a supply of bombykol was available through independent synthesis. Now, more than three decades after the structure of bombykol first became known, we have a large fund of information about this system in *Bombyx*. There have been enormous advances in molecular biology during this period, and the application of new methods has led to knowledge that was beyond conception when Butenandt began his pioneering effort. In 1989, for example, scientists learned the chemical structure of the peptide hormone in the brain of the silkworm moth that activates the moth's synthesis of bombykol. We also know the structure of the analogous hormone in the corn earworm *Heliothis zea*, a related moth. The two hormones are very similar. These findings in turn open new questions for research. How does this hormone deliver its message to produce bombykol? Is the corn earworm responsive to the related peptide from the silkworm moth?

Determination of the structure of bombykol also aroused immediate interest in learning about the chemistry of other pheromones. Here was a new area of research that

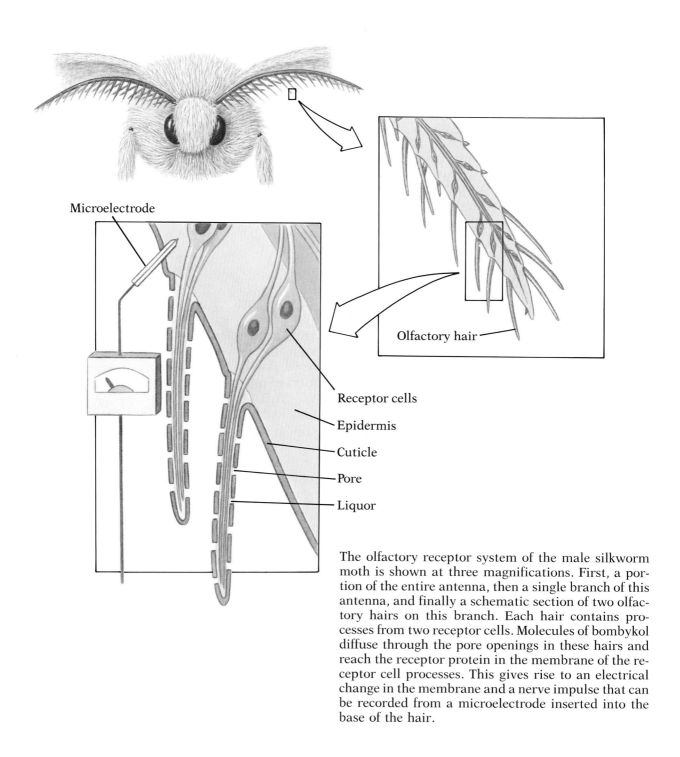

Microelectrode

Receptor cells

Epidermis

Cuticle

Pore

Liquor

Olfactory hair

The olfactory receptor system of the male silkworm moth is shown at three magnifications. First, a portion of the entire antenna, then a single branch of this antenna, and finally a schematic section of two olfactory hairs on this branch. Each hair contains processes from two receptor cells. Molecules of bombykol diffuse through the pore openings in these hairs and reach the receptor protein in the membrane of the receptor cell processes. This gives rise to an electrical change in the membrane and a nerve impulse that can be recorded from a microelectrode inserted into the base of the hair.

combined chemical techniques of isolation and structural elucidation with behavioral and biological studies. Attention soon widened from insects to other organisms, and with time improved techniques for such investigations emerged and became widely familiar. The enthusiastic explorations that began with the determination of the structure of bombykol have evolved into our present store of information on pheromonal chemistry in species from microbes to mammals.

Courting with Toxins

There is a group of butterflies called danaids that engage in an odd courtship ritual. The males have two brushlike structures, known as hairpencils, that are ordinarily tucked into the rear of the abdomen. In courtship these hairpencils emerge, and the male brushes their bristle-covered tips against the female. If the female finds this intimacy acceptable, she is then willing to mate with the male. Several research groups have contributed to our knowledge of mate selection by danaid butterflies, but we owe much of our insight here to Thomas Eisner and Jerrold Meinwald, biologist and chemist, respectively, at Cornell University. They and their research groups are responsible for many important advances of the past quarter century, both in pheromonal communication and also in the broader area of chemical ecology, which includes chemical interactions of all sorts within and among various species.

From the hairpencils of two species of danaids, *Lycorea ceres*, from Trinidad, and *Danaus gilippus*, the queen butterfly from Florida, Eisner and Meinwald were able to isolate and identify a surprising substance, a nitrogen-containing compound they named

Danaidone

danaidone. Danaidone does not look like any other pheromone that we have discussed. In fact, there is really only one group of natural substances that danaidone resembles structurally: some compounds found in several species of flowering plants and known as pyrrolizidine alkaloids. Pyrrolizidine is the chemical name of the general structural type of these compounds, and alkaloid is a generic designation for nitrogen-containing compounds derived from plants. The chemical resemblance of danaidone to these alkaloids suggested that perhaps the pheromone is derived from a food source of the butterfly. That is, perhaps the butterfly ingests these alkaloids in its regular diet of plant juices and then synthesizes its pheromone from them.

Microscopic examination of the hairpencils of *Danaus* revealed that its bristles were covered with tiny powdery particles carrying pheromone. During courtship the male dusts these particles onto the female's antennae, in this way transferring danaidone directly to her. The Cornell scientists first isolated danaidone as one of the principal components of hairpencils, without using a bioassay to determine its biological activity. They had deciphered its structure before demonstrating its function, but eventually they provided dramatic proof that danaidone is a pheromone.

Male *Danaus* butterflies raised in the laboratory are not successful in courting females. These males pursue females and waft their hairpencils over the antennae of females, just as wild males do, but they are only about 20 percent as likely as wild males to be accepted

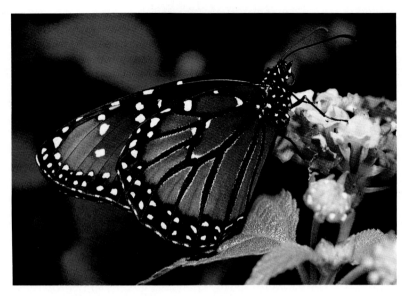 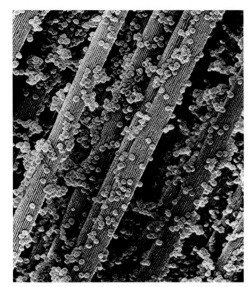

Left: An adult queen butterfly on a flower. *Right:* A scanning electron micrograph shows particles covered with pheromone clinging to hairs from a hairpencil of the queen butterfly.

by a female. Chemical analysis showed that the laboratory males carried virtually no danaidone. If natural or synthetic danaidone, dissolved in a little mineral oil, was applied to the hairpencils of these deficient males, they became as acceptable to females as wild butterflies.

The pheromone does come from pyrrolizidine alkaloids in the diet of the butterflies. In the wild, adult male danaids feed on fluids from plants containing the alkaloids, and it was the lack of this natural food source that left the laboratory-raised danaids without danaidone and inadequate. If laboratory danaids are given the alkaloids in their diet, they can convert these compounds to danaidone just as well as their wild relatives. They will even eat the pure compounds. If presented with a tiny crystal of a pyrrolizidine alkaloid,

a male *Danaus* will regurgitate a bit of fluid to dissolve the crystal and then imbibe the solution that is formed.

These butterflies seek out and eat plants containing these alkaloids preferentially. Yet, pyrrolizidine alkaloids are toxic to vertebrates and are avoided by other insects. It is generally thought that they protect the plants from most herbivores, which learn to avoid eating plants containing the alkaloids. Danaid butterflies appear to have borrowed the toxic alkaloids for their own protection. Besides serving as the raw material for synthesis of a pheromone, these compounds have another important role in the butterfly's reproductive biology. Males convert only a small portion of the alkaloids that they ingest to danaidone, storing about 80 percent of this toxic material unchanged in small sacs known as reproductive accessory glands. During copulation a male transfers the toxic alkaloids from these glands to the female. In turn, the female incorporates the alkaloids into her eggs, where they act to discourage predation. Beetles that prey on butterfly eggs avoid eating those that contain these alkaloids. From a toxin that protects plants, these butterflies have evolved a safeguard for their eggs.

The pheromone danaidone provides the receptive female a needed signal in her selection of a mate, and Eisner and Meinwald have suggested that the pheromone actually gives the female critical information about her suitor. Their proposal is that during courtship the female judges the male's store of toxic alkaloids by the amount of pheromone he has available to dust over her. A male that showers a heavy dose of danaidone on a female is saying that he can present her a generous nuptial gift of alkaloids. The female should prefer this male. The more toxin the male can donate, the more she can put into her eggs, and the better their chance of survival. Experiments have shown that the amount of pheromone in a male does reflect quantitatively his store of defensive alkaloids, in line with the idea Eisner and Meinwald put forward. One question for the future is whether the male can cheat. Do some males have a way to promise more defensive toxins than they can deliver, or are they always honest butterflies?

The male *Danaus* has overcome a defensive mechanism of plants that contain pyrrolizidine alkaloids, and he preferentially feeds on these species. Evolution has turned these toxins to the butterfly's own purposes, and, according to Eisner and Meinwald's suggestion, has fashioned an indicator for his potential mate of his supply of the alkaloids. Similar mechanisms are probably at work in some related species.

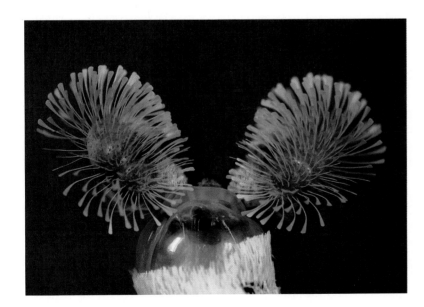

The hairpencils of a male *Utetheisa ornatrix*. Although this common Caribbean moth is not a close relative of the danaid butterflies, it has a related pheromone with a similar delivery system. Just like male danaids, the male moth synthesizes the pheromone from pyrrolizidine alkaloids in his diet and transfers this signal to the female during courtship.

A Summoning of Beetles

Danaid butterflies obtain the raw materials for their pyrrolizidine pheromones from plants. In a similar manner, bark beetles use compounds from their hosts to make aggregation pheromones. Bark beetles are small insects, some no more than 2 millimeters (0.08 inch) long. They invade trees, bore into the wood, and breed. There are many species, and we are concerned particularly with ones that rapidly aggregate in large numbers on their host, in what is called a mass attack. Some of these beetles assault living trees, some favor weak or dying trees, and still others breed in recently fallen timber. In a nice example of insect specialization, the site of breeding within a tree may also vary from species to species. There are some that prefer the upper trunk, some the lower trunk, and some the crown of the tree. In this way several kinds of beetle that specialize in the same host species can coexist on a single tree without stressful competition.

A mass attack by these beetles commences with one insect landing on a potential host. If its initial investigation is favorable, this pioneer is soon joined by more beetles, and these by still more. They bore into the wood and form galleries where the females lay their eggs. When the eggs hatch, the larvae feed on the wood and burrow further into the surrounding tissue. At the end of the galleries, the larvae pupate and undergo metamorphosis into adults. The new adults emerge, tunnel out through the bark, and fly away to seek new trees.

The aggregation and breeding of large numbers of beetles can overwhelm and kill a healthy tree. Several species of these insects are a continuing menace to both timber and shade trees. Two species (*Scolytus scolytus* and *Scolytus multistriatus*) carry the fungus *Ceratocystis ulmi* that causes Dutch elm dis-

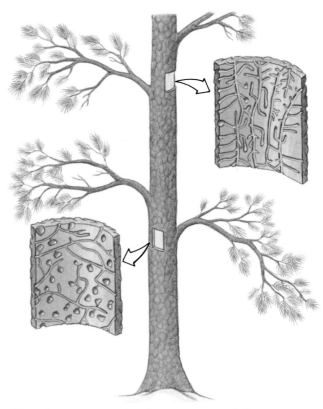

The pine engraver beetle *Ips pini* and the Southern pine beetle *Dendroctonus frontalis* both attack large pine trees, but they prefer different parts of the tree. *I. pini* bores its galleries in the top of the tree, while *D. frontalis* colonizes the middle and lower trunk.

ease. The economic importance of these beetles has provided the practical impetus for careful examination of the chemistry and biology of their aggregation. Chemical communication orchestrates the destructive mass attacks of these pests, and effective manipulation and control of their signals would be an attractive way to manage them.

We will now consider the events leading to aggregation in greater detail. Because several species of bark beetle may occupy the same territory and may interact in important ways, our discussion here covers more than one species and its pheromones.

The first event in aggregation is the landing of one beetle on a host tree. In some cases the beetle has been lured by chemicals emitted by the tree that mark it as an attractive host. Under some conditions, for example, ethanol is released as dying trees decompose. The ambrosia beetle *Trypodendron lineatum* detects this ethanol and homes in on its target. Other species of beetle appear to light on trees at random, deciding only after landing, and possibly boring into the wood, whether the tree deserves further attention. Perhaps the tree is the wrong species or is somehow resistant to colonization. A healthy flow of resin in response to a test boring may flush the beetle from its hole and lead to its retreat. The beetle may move to a less resistant host.

Once a beetle has settled on an appropriate tree, it sends out a pheromone that draws others to its find. The sex of the initial explorer depends on the species and its habits. In polygamous species males strike first, and each arriving male initiates his own attack on the tree. As females arrive, they locate holes bored by the males, enter, mate with the resident males, and then construct galleries where their eggs are laid. Several females may enter and mate with a single male in the hole he has made. In monogamous species, females are generally the first to arrive. In each case, the first wave of arriving beetles starts producing the aggregation pheromone as it takes up the assault. The signal grows stronger with each new arrival, and more join the call until the host is fully colonized.

Nearby trees may be caught in the onslaught as beetles drawn to the area land on them as well, and this can lead to a cluster of killed trees. Such spreading of a mass attack to neighboring trees results in some cases from an extraordinary feature of the pheromonal response. For some species the concentration

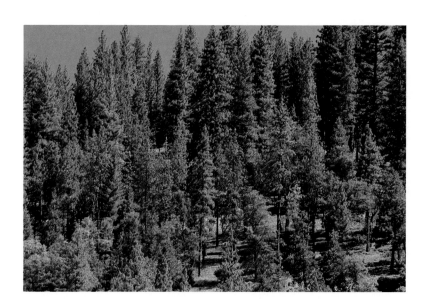

A group of pine trees killed by an infestation of bark beetles in the El Dorado National Forest, California.

Peeling away the bark of a pondorosa pine reveals an adult *Ips paraconfusus* clearing frass from its gallery. The small side channels contain feeding larvae.

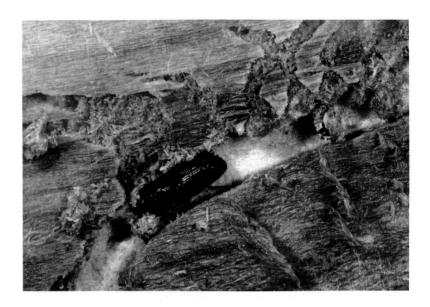

of pheromone toward which the beetles are drawn has an upper limit. Above this limit, they no longer move toward the source but rather land on a nearby tree and launch their offensive there. The original tree can support only so many beetles, and this simple mechanism discourages too many from colonizing a single host.

We owe the first chemical identification of a beetle aggregation pheromone to R. M. Silverstein, a chemist at the College of Environmental Science and Forestry of the State University of New York, and D. L. Wood, an entomologist at the University of California at Berkeley, who examined the California five-spined engraver beetle *Ips paraconfusus*. *I. paraconfusus* feeds on ponderosa pine *Pinus ponderosa*, and as the male bores and eats, he creates boring dust and expels feces from his hindgut. The feces contain the pheromone, and the entire mixture of feces, dust, and pheromone that piles up behind the boring beetle is known as frass.

In the mid-1960s Silverstein, Wood, and their co-workers collected several kilograms of frass, extracted it with organic solvent, and fractionated the extract. They monitored their isolation with a bioassay in which beetles walked upwind toward the sources of the odors. The walking bioassay proved to be more easily managed than one that required the beetles to fly to the pheromone, as they do in nature. This study identified the pheromone that causes *I. paraconfusus* to aggregate as a mixture of three components: ipsenol, ipsdienol, and *cis*-verbenol. The three compounds act synergistically; separately, none of them is particularly efficacious. Thanks to improved techniques, scientists no longer have to extract mountains of frass in order to obtain beetle attractants; they can now collect pheromones directly from the air surrounding the actively boring beetles.

Ponderosa pine produces two compounds called myrcene and α-pinene. The male beetle takes these compounds from the host tree as

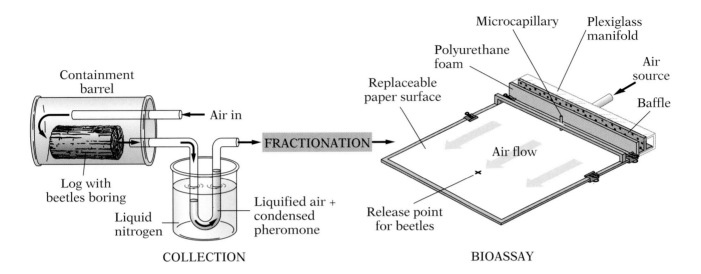

To identify bark beetle aggregation pheromones, investigators liquified all the volatile compounds produced by beetles boring in a log and then fractionated the concentrated material by gas chromatography. They tested the attractivity of each fraction by observing whether beetles would walk upwind toward the odor source on the flat bed of the bioassay apparatus. This bed was covered with a sheet of paper that could be replaced after each test so that the apparatus would not be contaminated by pheromones released during the bioassay.

With the aid of bacteria, the male *Ips paraconfusus* converts myrcene and α-pinene into its aggregation pheromones.

starting materials for the pheromone, and then enlists the assistance of bacteria in carrying out the chemical transformations. Myrcene seems to be converted to ipsenol and ipsdienol by the bacterium *Bacillus cereus* that makes its home in the hindgut of *I. paraconfusus*. The isolated bacterium can convert myrcene to ipsenol and ipsdienol, and *α*-pinene to *cis*-verbenol. Male beetles that were first treated with the antibiotic streptomycin produced no ipsenol or ipsdienol after ingesting myrcene. Because streptomycin kills *B. cereus*, this result indicates that it is the gut bacteria that produce the pheromone. Surprisingly, the antibiotic did not suppress the synthesis of *cis*-verbenol, so perhaps both the beetle and the bacterium can perform this transformation.

The western pine beetle *Dendroctonus brevicomis* also colonizes ponderosa pine, and this species makes direct use of the myrcene produced by the tree as an ingredient of its aggregation pheromone. The Silverstein and Wood team also identified the constituents of this pheromone. In this monogamous beetle the female arrives first and begins to emit a blend of myrcene taken up from the host tree and *exo*-brevicomin, a compound that she makes. This mixture attracts male beetles preferentially, and they discharge a third compound, frontalin, at the entrance of the holes bored by the females.

The mixture of brevicomin, myrcene, and frontalin now lures males and females equally. As more beetles arrive, both males and females now start to release *trans*-verbenol and verbenone, a combination that inhibits further response to the pheromone. This third signal has the same effect as the upper-limit concentration of aggregation pheromone mentioned above. In this way the established *D. brevicomis* direct late-arriving beetles to alternative hosts and avoid overcrowding on the tree first attacked.

Messages That Reach Others

The aggregation pheromone brings more beetles of the same species from near and far to join in the raid, but these are not the only creatures to arrive. As many as one hundred different species of insects have been trapped on pine trees infested with *D. brevicomis*. These included predaceous beetles and flies, some of which feed on larval bark beetles, some on adults. In several cases, these enemies are drawn specifically to the bark beetle pheromone. One of these is *Temnochila chlorodia*, a beetle that feeds on adult bark beetles. In addition, it lays its eggs on infested trees so that its larvae will be near their prey, which is the bark beetle brood. In a field test of a mixture of *exo*-brevicomin, frontalin, and myrcene as a bark beetle attractant, large numbers of both bark beetles and *T. chlorodia* were attracted and trapped. The situation is complex, however, and cues other than aggregation pheromones can also be important. For example, some species that prey on bark beetles are attracted by volatile compounds emitted by the host tree under siege.

The pheromonal message also reaches other kinds of bark beetles living in the same area. Sometimes these other beetles are able to turn this information to their own use. *Ips paraconfusus* and *Ips pini* live together in northern California, where both strike ponderosa pine. When the two species are present on a single host, it appears that neither one can make efficient use of the space. They somehow interfere with each other. Their galleries are unevenly distributed, and the consequence is a reduction in brood for both species. Both beetles suffer, for there are fewer progeny than there might have been. It is an obvious advantage for *I. paraconfusus* and *I. pini* to steer clear of each other's trees. Neither species responds to the aggregation pheromone of the

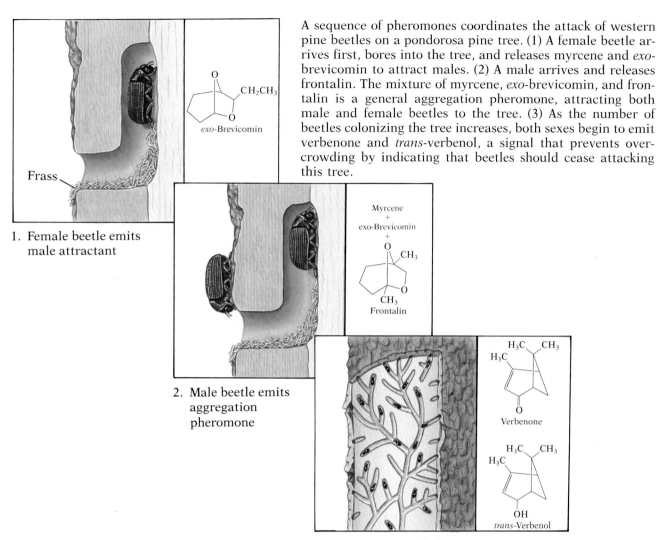

A sequence of pheromones coordinates the attack of western pine beetles on a pondorosa pine tree. (1) A female beetle arrives first, bores into the tree, and releases myrcene and *exo*-brevicomin to attract males. (2) A male arrives and releases frontalin. The mixture of myrcene, *exo*-brevicomin, and frontalin is a general aggregation pheromone, attracting both male and female beetles to the tree. (3) As the number of beetles colonizing the tree increases, both sexes begin to emit verbenone and *trans*-verbenol, a signal that prevents overcrowding by indicating that beetles should cease attacking this tree.

1. Female beetle emits male attractant

2. Male beetle emits aggregation pheromone

3. Beetles on crowded tree emit aggregation inhibitors

other, but there is a further, more subtle interaction that helps keep them apart.

Each aggregation pheromone not only attracts members of the emitting species, but it also repels the other species. If many *I. pini* and a few *I. paraconfusus* are broadcasting their two pheromones from a single host tree,

the stronger *I. pini* signal prevents distant *I. paraconfusus* from responding to their own pheromone. Consequently, most beetles arriving at the tree will be *I. pini*. This blocking effect probably involves central processing of signals in the brain rather than any competitive interaction of distinct pheromones at receptors in the antennae. There are several other instances of interspecific effects of pheromones in bark beetles, some involving as many as four different species. Responses may be mutually enhanced, rather than blocked, if two species can profitably share separate parts of the same host.

These are examples of pheromones that disclose information not only within a species, but also to other species. Our original definition did not cover this complication. We spoke earlier of pheromones as signals originating with an organism and bearing a message to other members of its species, but these bark beetle signals do more than that. As we learn more about chemical interactions among organisms, our former neat and simple definition requires qualification. We have also come to expect compounds to be specifically synthesized by organisms for their role as pheromones. We have seen here, however, that *D. brevicomis* makes use of an unmodified host chemical, myrcene, as a constituent of its aggregation pheromone. An earlier example of the same phenomenon was cholesteryl oleate, which is ingested and excreted by several ticks as a mounting pheromone. More complications will appear below, and many more doubtless remain to be discovered.

We may hope someday to control forest pests by manipulating aggregation signals, but for now a large-scale undertaking is not practical. We still do not have a complete grasp of the multiple interactions among the species. Chemicals that interrupt the aggregation response have been used to deter bark beetles in several instances, and, as we note in the next section, there have been trial trappings of some species on a large scale. There is still a long way to go, however, before aggregation pheromones become a routine tool for managing forest pests.

Toward the Use of Pheromones in Pest Control

Perhaps pheromones will provide the means for controlling bark beetles in the future, but reaching that goal depends on understanding complex ecological and economic considerations. It is now time for us to look at the matter of pest control in more detail. After all, it is the prospect of applying our knowledge to agriculture and forestry that has paid the bill for much of our present knowledge about chemical communication. How has this investment paid off? In general, pheromones have found three types of application in pest control.

The first and currently most important of these applications is the use of natural attractants as a convenient analytical tool for estimating insect populations. Traps are set out baited with the attractant pheromone of a particular pest, and from the numbers of individuals lured and caught in these traps, the total population of the insect in the area can be extrapolated. With this knowledge, farmers can adjust the spraying of insecticides or the use of other control measures for maximum positive effect. Especially important, they can limit the use of insecticides to the shortest possible time. In the same way, monitoring of a pest population after control measures permits evaluation of their success. The trapping technique can also serve as a critical early warning device. The Mediterranean fruit fly *Ceratitis capitata* was introduced accidentally into California in 1980 with disastrous effects on the state's agriculture. Its presence there was first detected in traps baited with a pheromone synthesized in the laboratory. Governmental agencies regularly monitor local populations of several exotic insect pests in

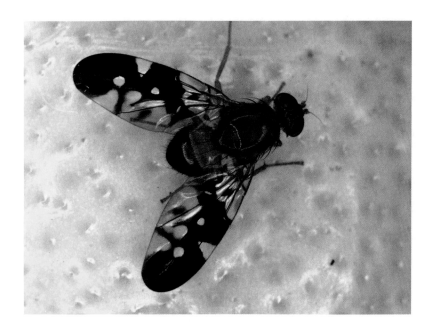

A Mediterranean fruit fly, or medfly, which is an established insect pest in many parts of the world. Continuing surveillance by some 40,000 early-warning traps, located mainly in Florida and California, has prevented this insect from becoming permanently established in the United States. An incipient infestation detected in Los Angeles in 1987 cost two million dollars to eradicate.

this fashion, particularly in Florida, Texas, and California.

A second practical use of pheromones in pest control is a simple conceptual extension of the trapping of a representative sample. With enough traps, perhaps all of a local population, or of one sex, of a pest could be trapped and its life cycle broken. This trap-out strategy, as it is called, would seem to hold promise for bark beetles, since they aggregate naturally in large numbers. The idea is simply to replace trees with traps at the site of aggregation. An extensive trap-out program of this sort was undertaken in Norway and Sweden in 1979, following an explosion in the population of the spruce beetle *Ips typographus*. The threat to the vast Scandinavian spruce forests was severe, and to counter it, 600,000 baited pheromone traps were prepared and distributed throughout the infested woodlands of the

two countries. These traps captured nearly three thousand million beetles in 1979 and nearly four thousand million the next year. Despite the success in eliminating such huge numbers of beetles, the infestation was devastating and led to a ruinous loss of trees. Whether it would have been even worse without the trapping program is uncertain.

The third application of chemical signals is known as mating disruption. The concept is not unlike that of radio jamming, in which a powerful interfering signal is broadcast to block reception on a particular wavelength. In the same way, spreading an attractant pheromone throughout a crop area should impair the ability of an insect to locate prospective mates that are emitting the same pheromone. Investigators have discovered that several species of insects respond to an attractant by flying upwind in a zigzag pattern within the

This commercial monitoring trap in an orange tree releases an attractant of the citrus cutworm *Xylomyges curialis.* Moths drawn to the trap are caught on its sticky inside surface and can then be counted. Citrus cutworm is an erratic pest that does not strike every year but can be a problem in the citrus groves of central and southern California. Monitoring traps alert growers to its arrival.

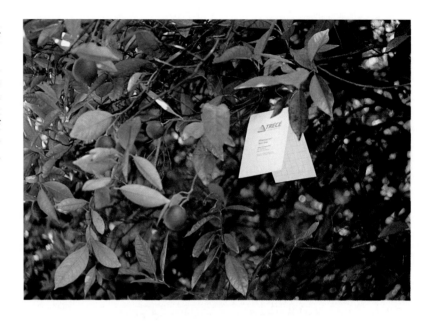

spreading airborne signal. Ordinarily, this behavior leads efficiently to a mate. However, when many artificial sources are emitting the pheromone in a crop area, flying upwind need not lead to a mate at all. Because pheromones function in such low concentrations and are so specific in their action, the idea has long been an appealing approach to pest control.

In typical field applications, the disrupting pheromone is dispersed either aerially or from dispensers scattered throughout the crop area. In the latter case, many insects are naturally attracted directly to the dispensers, and this approach takes on characteristics of the trap-out strategy. This situation has led workers to modify the mating disruption strategy by adding an insecticide to the pheromone in the dispenser, creating an "attracticide." Not only does the high level of pheromone in the field interfere with mate location, but many insects are killed outright at the dispensers. One of the objectionable side effects of spraying with insecticides is that beneficial insects are inevi-

tably destroyed along with the targeted pest. In several cases the attracticide technique has permitted farmers to use an insecticide against a pest effectively without wholesale elimination of useful species from the area.

One Triumph

Mating disruption is the technique responsible for what is probably the most successful commercial use of a pheromone against an agricultural pest that has yet been carried out. The pink bollworm *Pectinophora gossypiella* causes serious losses of cotton (*Gossypium herbaceum* and related species) in the United States. In 1977, H. H. Shorey and his research group in the Department of Entomology of the University of California at Riverside, together with a group led by T. W. Brooks at Conrel, then a division of the Albany International Company, demonstrated the feasibility of using the pink bollworm attractant pheromone for disruption of mating in field tests. This attractant, known as gossyplure, is discharged by the female and is a 60:40 mixture of two compounds that differ only by the arrangement of the groups about one double bond. These successful field tests came at a time of general disappointment with pheromones, which had not lived up to their earlier promise for practical insect control.

The following year gossyplure was registered by the Environmental Protection Agency as the first approved mating disruptant. The EPA's action and Shorey's and Brook's reports raised spirits and gave strong encouragement to research on pheromones at a difficult time. However, both technical and practical considerations hampered widespread adoption of this new methodology. Skeptics questioned whether the method really worked, and critics complained that adequate control experiments were lacking. There were the difficulties of convincing individual cotton growers to replace familiar insecticides with this novel approach to pest control. There was the implicit threat to the insecticide industry.

Something finally happened to push these reservations aside. After being a problem in the southeastern United States and Texas for some years, pink bollworm reached the irrigated cotton fields of southern California in 1966. By 1980 cotton yields in southern California's Imperial Valley had declined by 35 percent from their level in the early 1960s despite increasingly heavy use of insecticides. Two sprayings per season were normal before 1965, but by 1980, ten to fifteen were necessary. The increase reflected not only an expanding population of pink bollworm, but also the bollworm's ever-growing resistance to the insecticides deployed against it. These broad-spectrum toxins destroy beneficial insects along with unwanted pests. In 1981 this unavoidable side effect led to disaster when a severe infestation of the whitefly *Bemesia tabacci* struck the cotton fields. This pest is normally kept well under control by natural insect predators, but the numbers of those predators had been much diminished by the repeated sprayings for pink bollworm. Whitefly not only lowers the yield of cotton, but it also reduces the quality and value of the fiber by contaminating it with whitefly honeydew, turning it into what is called "sticky cotton." In addition, fruit and vegetable crops in neighboring fields

Glossyplure is a mixture of these two compounds, 60 percent of the top one and 40 percent of the bottom one. The two compounds differ only in the position of attachment of the $CH_3CH_2CH_2CH_2—$ group to one of the double bonds.

A mature pink bollworm in a damaged boll of cotton. This "worm" is the larva of the moth *Pectinophora gossypiella,* which is regarded as one of the most destructive insects in the world.

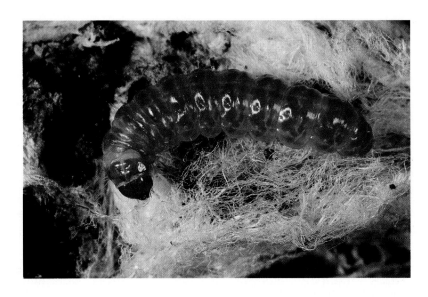

were devastated by a viral disease carried by the whitefly.

In response to this disaster, the cotton growers of the Imperial Valley agreed to establish a legally constituted pest abatement district with mandated sprayings of gossyplure for 1982. Under this arrangement all 18,226 hectares (just over 45,000 acres) of the Imperial Valley planted to cotton received at least four sprayings of the pheromone for mating disruption early in the 1982 growing season, after which growers were free either to continue with the pheromone or to switch to their familiar insecticides. The goal of the program was to minimize application of insecticdes until August 1982 and thus prevent recurrence of the whitefly infestation of 1981. The program was carried out successfully, and it largely accomplished its purposes. The whitefly problem did not recur, and beneficial insects were maintained in the fields well into August. The yield of cotton was up 24 percent over its 1981 level, and pink bollworm was down. The pheromone treatment had cost about the same as spraying with broad-spectrum insecticides.

There were no control plots, because the abatement district comprised all cotton fields in the valley. However, a separate growing area 120 miles away that received conventional treatment with insecticides that year had a cotton yield only 73 percent as great as the valley. In this second area the level of pink bollworm larval infestation was 32.6 percent, while in the valley it was only 5.8 percent.

The abatement district was not renewed for the 1983 growing season, because growers preferred to reassert individual choice over pest control. Nonetheless, in 1983 most cotton acreage in the valley received voluntary treatment with gossyplure early in the season. By 1989, the pheromone in various formulations was widely used for control of pink bollworm in southern California, although the number of acres in the area planted to cotton had declined more than 40 percent since 1982. The opinion of observers at the University of California and the U.S. Department of Agriculture is that these efforts in the Imperial Valley have been successful and that use of gossyplure and other pheromones will increase in future programs of integrated pest management for cotton and other crops.

The achievement with gossyplure is unsurpassed in terms of grower acceptance and acreage treated. While it has demonstrated that mating disruption is practical on a large scale, this experience has also disclosed numerous obstacles to the translation of an orderly scientific protocol into a workable agricultural procedure. One part of the problem is a mismatch between the inherent characteristics of pheromones and the needs and interests of the chemical industry that must manufacture the formulations for field use. To many scientists working to create a replacement for conventional insecticides, pheromonal control of pests offers an elegant and intellectually appealing solution to an increasingly urgent environmental problem. A tiny amount of a relatively simple, natural compound acts against an insect enemy without disrupting other species or incurring great environmental cost. A carefully aimed magic bullet replaces the sweeping fire of a machine gun.

Regrettably, these very characteristics contribute to a lack of commercial interest in pheromones. Natural compounds cannot themselves be patented. Different pests require different pheromones, so diverse compounds and multiple formulations are needed. Pheromones are effective in relatively small amounts, so large-scale production of these substances is not foreseen. In contrast, new broad-spectrum insecticides are typically patentable and needed in large quantities, and one agent is effective against many different pests.

This is only one of the complex problems that have impeded the introduction of pheromones into agriculture. There are also bureaucratic, political, technical, and economic hurdles, and so far the pace of change has been discouragingly slow. The first serious suggestion that insect attractants could offer a practical means of controlling agricultural pests came from Bruno Götz in 1939 following his extensive experimentation with the grape vine moth *Lobesia botrana* in German vineyards. The American public's awareness of the issues surrounding increasing use of insecticides dates from the publication in 1962 of Rachel Carson's *Silent Spring*. We have just seen that to the present the most successful commercial experience with a pheromone for pest control concerned about 45,000 acres of cotton in 1982. Perhaps the pace will quicken.

Spiders That Mimic a Moth's Sex Attractant

The attraction of several different species to bark beetle aggregation pheromones shows that the role of chemical signals can be complicated. Another complication that we must consider is pheromone mimicry. Some organisms have developed an ability to imitate signals used by others and turn them to their own advantage. Investigations by William G. Eberhard of the Universidad del Valle in Colombia have provided a remarkable example of pheromone mimicry in spiders of the genus *Mastophora*.

These spiders are known as bolas spiders. Females do not weave webs but instead collect their freshly spun silk into a sticky ball and hang it from a vertical line attached to a single horizontal line. At night when a bolas spider is ready to "hunt," she hangs from the horizontal line near the ball. Using her front legs, she grasps the vertical line above the ball. By pulling on this line, she can move the ball. She then begins to emit a volatile signal that mimics the sex attractant of the fall armyworm *Spodoptera frugiperda*, a common local moth. Downwind, a male moth responds to the attractant and flies toward the waiting spider. As he comes within range, the spider swings the ball at him. If she hits him, the ball sticks to the moth and he is caught. The spider descends the line, paralyzes the moth, and feeds on him at her leisure. This unlikely method of hunting turns out to be competitive with the techniques of web-building spiders. Eberhard found that a hunting bolas spider attracted a moth about every six minutes. Most of these did not come close enough to be swung at, and the spider swung at others and missed. On average, however, a spider got about 2.2 moths for a night of hunting, or about 18 percent of her body weight per day. This rate of predation compares well with that of conventional web spiders.

No chemist has analyzed the bolas spider's signal, but we can suspect that the spider has evolved a way to synthesize the same com-

pounds that make up the fall armyworm's attractant. Pheromone mimicry indicates that, as with codes and ciphers, leaks can occur in the signalling system. Outsiders may steal crucial information and turn it against the intended recipients.

Orchids That Seduce Bees and Wasps

A group of orchids that depend on insects for their fertilization practice a different sort of pheromone mimicry. Many kinds of flowers contain a drop of nectar that attracts hungry insects. In collecting this bit of food, a visiting insect picks up pollen that it then transfers to other flowers, pollinating them as it continues foraging. Instead of encouraging insects with food, however, some orchids appear to offer sex. Several groups of Mediterranean and South American orchids have flowers with

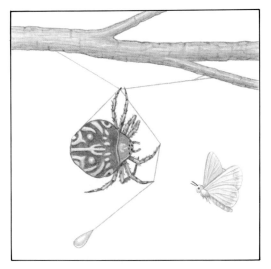 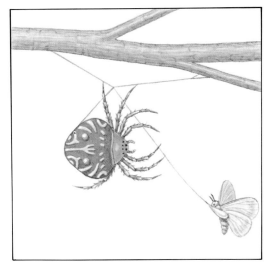

A bolas spider captures a meal by swinging her sticky ball of silk and hitting a male fall armyworm moth.

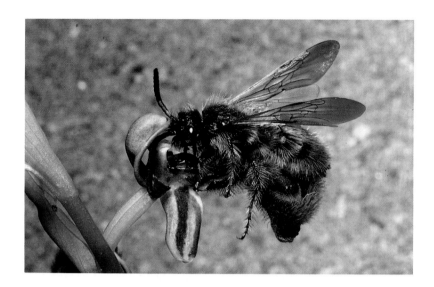

The western Mediterranean orchid *Ophrys speculum* emits a scent that attracts the burrowing wasp *Campsoscolia ciliata*, which here is pseudocopulating with an orchid flower. Normally the male wasps emerge about a month before the females, and during this period the males pollinate the orchid. In years when the female wasps emerge early or the plant blooms late, few orchid seeds are formed.

parts that closely resemble the female of a local bee or wasp. The male insects are deceived by this similarity and attempt to copulate with the flower. During this "pseudocopulation," the male picks up pollen, which he carries to his next encounter with a flower. This deception is successful in part because male bees emerge earlier than females in many species, and the orchids are ready for pollination when there are many male bees but few females. The male bees begin to neglect the orchids when the females emerge, but by that time the main flowering season has usually ended.

Orchids of the genus *Ophrys* that grow around the Mediterranean have improved upon this deceptive scheme. These flowers broadcast scents that imitate the sex pheromones of the insects they resemble. Some attract a single species; others have a wider appeal, often enticing several related bees or wasps. A chemical signal can lure male insects from afar and thus better the orchids' chances of pollination.

Complex Signals in a Complex Society

Chemical communication probably reaches its greatest refinement in the social insects. These are the ants, termites, and social bees and wasps, and it would be possible to devote a small book to the chemical signals of each of them. These creatures lead complex lives with remarkable divisions of labor. There are sometimes thousands of individuals that must continually be guided, instructed, and encouraged in the many activities required to maintain an elaborate community. Nurses, undertakers, food gatherers, soldiers, and other castes have their duties, and the messages to manage these endeavors must pass from one member of the colony to another, often in the darkness of an underground or enclosed nest. Some of these signals trigger immediate behavioral reactions; others evoke physiological changes. Some act to block reactions or changes. That is, there is no reaction or change as long as the pheromone is present; but if the signal vanishes, the insects react or change physiologically. E. O. Wilson and Bert Hölldobler, two renowned authorities on ants who were both at Harvard University at the time, have estimated that the operation of an ant colony demands ten to twenty kinds of signals and that most of these are chemical signals. More than thirty pheromonal signals have been identified in the honey bee, which is the most extensively studied of the social insects. We shall consider the honey bee in some detail and then discuss a few pheromones found in ants.

The admired industry of the common honey bee is under the strict control of chemical signals. Pheromones govern food gathering, brood rearing, colony growth and defense, and reproduction. Deprived of continual signals on these vital topics, life in the beehive soon loses its natural order and efficiency. Many research groups, motivated by both practical needs and scientific curiosity, have contributed to our knowledge of these activities in the lives of bees, but the story is complex and still far from complete. Not only is the pheromone that transmits a particular message a mixture of chemicals, but the same chemicals appear repeatedly, delivering diverse messages as the context changes. We know the identity of only a fraction of the compounds in these pheromones. Several glands contribute to these signals, but for some of these glands we cannot even specify the major constituents of their secretions. At the other extreme, more than a dozen compounds have been identified in a particular gland of the queen bee, but it is not yet clear what role, if any, most of them play in the queen's stream of messages to her colony. Another complication challenging scientists is that honey bees can distinguish whether certain signals come from their own hive or that of another colony. Pheromones composed of mixtures of compounds offer an easy way to differentiate the signals of one colony from those of another. The composition of a multicomponent signal may be slightly varied to indicate its source without changing the message.

Queen Pheromone

In a colony of honey bees the pheromone with the broadest effect is emitted by the queen and spread throughout the colony by workers. When a queen is present, a colony is stable and cohesive. If the queen is removed, social conditions quickly deteriorate. When she is not moving about, the queen is constantly surrounded by an ever-changing court of six to eight workers who continually lick her and examine her with their antennae. In the course of their ministrations the courtiers pick up queen pheromone from her body. The maintenance of stability depends on workers who withdraw from the queen's court and circulate throughout the hive with the information that the queen is indeed in place. They do this by passing the queen pheromone to other workers during the first several minutes after they leave the queen's presence. A bee that has recently been at court is particularly attractive to other workers, and they appear eager to interact with her.

Queen pheromone has a number of other functions. It attracts drones during a queen's mating flights and also governs reproduction. Larvae from fertilized eggs can develop into either workers or queens, depending on how the nurse bees care for them. When the workers no longer receive an adequate amount of queen pheromone, they build queen cells and embark on the process of rearing new queens. This can happen when the queen reaches an advanced age or is removed from the colony, or when the hive grows too large or crowded for the queen pheromone to reach all its mem-

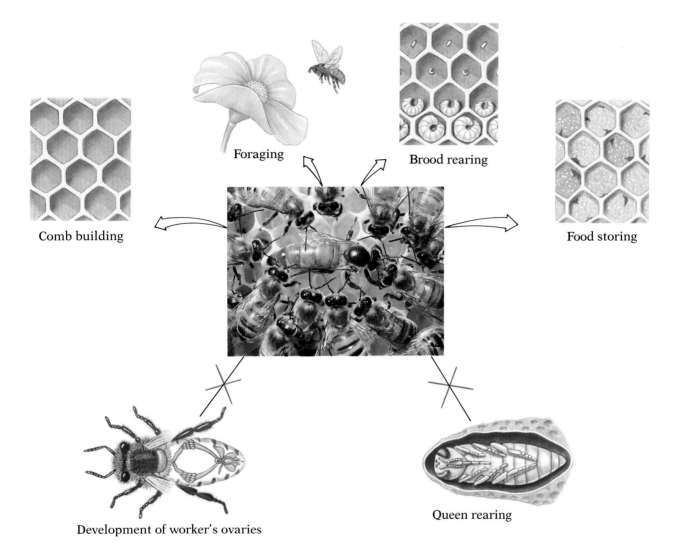

Comb building

Foraging

Brood rearing

Food storing

Development of worker's ovaries

Queen rearing

This court of worker honey bees around the queen changes members continually. Bees spend a few minutes at court, pick up queen pheromone, and then spread it throughout the hive. An adequate amount of queen pheromone keeps the workers at the many tasks necessary for a smoothly functioning colony. Presence of the pheromone also suppresses maturation of the workers' ovaries and inhibits the workers from rearing new queens.

bers. The workers refrain from building new queen cells as long as a healthy queen is in place and is providing enough queen pheromone for all. By producing an adequate supply of queen pheromone, a healthy queen forestalls the threat that would be posed by the emergence of new queens. A colony without a queen, however, is doomed. Without the stabilizing and organizing effects of queen pheromone, the colony soon disintegrates. This happens, for example, if there are no young larvae from which a new queen could be reared at the time the queen is lost. Here the queen pheromone governs reproduction in another way. The presence of queen pheromone suppresses development of the worker bees' ovaries, which remain immature. When a queen is lost, up to 25 percent of the workers undergo full maturation of their ovaries and start laying eggs.

Queen pheromone also stimulates workers to build new comb, rear more bees, forage, and store food. Without sufficient pheromonal stimulus, many workers will simply remain idle. The queen constantly disseminates a message that incites the rest of the community to selfless toil. Each colony has only one queen, and with a roughly constant rate of production of queen pheromone, we should expect the amount available to stimulate the labor of each worker to be greater in small colonies than in large ones. In fact, small colonies have a longer annual period of brood rearing and a higher rate of comb production per bee.

The queen pheromone that evokes these complex effects is a mixture of many chemical compounds. They come mainly from the mandibular glands, located in the queen's head, and the tergite glands, located in her abdomen. The most abundant compound in this mixture is able to induce the various effects of queen pheromone in tests carried out by several groups of scientists. In every investigation, however, it is less effective than the total natural mix of compounds.

Repellent Pheromone

The feces of virgin queens contain a specialized pheromone that serves to repel worker bees. A number of situations in the colony, such as the presence of an aging queen, motivate workers to raise queen larvae and permit several new virgin queens to emerge. When this happens, the queens fight until all but one of them has been stung and killed. During these deadly encounters the rival queens frequently eject fecal fluid that causes workers to move back and away from the arena of battle. Of the several compounds isolated from this fluid, only one of them efficiently repelled workers in a bioassay.

Nasonov Pheromone

The Nasonov gland develops only in worker bees. Neither drones nor queens have this gland, which is named after its nineteenth-century Russian discoverer. While emitting pheromone from this gland, the worker fans her wings to disperse it. Investigations at the beginning of the century showed that this

$$CH_3\overset{\overset{\displaystyle O}{\|}}{C}CH_2CH_2CH_2CH_2CH_2 \underset{H}{\overset{H}{\diagup}}C=C\underset{H}{\overset{\overset{\displaystyle O}{\|}}{\diagdown}COH}$$

The main component of queen pheromone. This carboxylic acid can evoke the responses of the pheromone but is less effective than the natural pheromone.

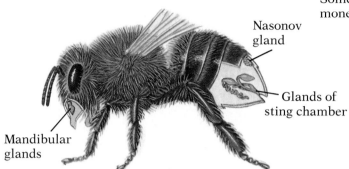

Some of the glands that produce and store pheromones in a worker honey bee.

Nasonov
gland

Glands of
sting chamber

Mandibular
glands

pheromone is an attractant, and it is now
clear that workers commonly release it in one
of three behavioral situations: when in a
swarm or forming a cluster, when marking the
entrance to their nest, or when indicating the
location of water on which they are foraging.

In swarming, a group of bees with a queen
leaves its parent colony and prepares to start
a new nest. The bees cluster on a support,
such as a tree branch, near the former hive.
The first bees to arrive emit Nasonov pheromone and bring other bees to their locale.
Scout bees then move out to seek a new permanent nesting site. Once they agree upon a
suitable spot, they return to the swarm and
disclose its location by performing a dance
that gives its direction and distance. Then they
return to the new site and release Nasonov
pheromone at its entrance. The swarm of bees
moves to the new location, and as the workers
walk in through the entrance, they too discharge Nasonov pheromone. A component of
queen pheromone also causes workers to release Nasonov pheromone. If, for example, the
queen is moved from a swarm to a position
nearby, workers in the swarm will soon dis-
cover her and liberate the signal in her vicin-

ity. Shortly the entire swarm joins the queen
in her new setting.

Bees at the entrance of an established nest
broadcast Nasonov pheromone to aid disoriented workers in finding their way home. They
fan the attractant away from the nest entrance, so that it becomes mixed with odors
from within and is presumably even more enticing. Nasonov pheromone not only attracts
bees, but also induces them to emit their own
Nasonov pheromone. As bees arrive at the entrance, they too send out the signal. Workers
also throng at the hive entrance and fill the
air with the pheromone during the queen's
mating flight, apparently helping her find her
way back after mating. Foraging workers emit
Nasonov pheromone to recruit nearby colleagues to a particularly rewarding site, usually a source of water rather than nectar or
pollen.

The secretion of the Nasonov gland contains seven closely related components. All of
these are well-known, fragrant compounds
from the essential oils of flowering plants, or
substances closely related to them. The components of Nasonov pheromone have all been
evaluated in diverse combinations in bioassays

When a colony grows so large that the bees are overcrowded, workers rear new queens. The old queen and about half of the bees leave the hive and form a swarm cluster on a nearby tree. This swarm, with the queen somewhere in the middle, waits for scouts to report the location of a suitable site for their new colony.

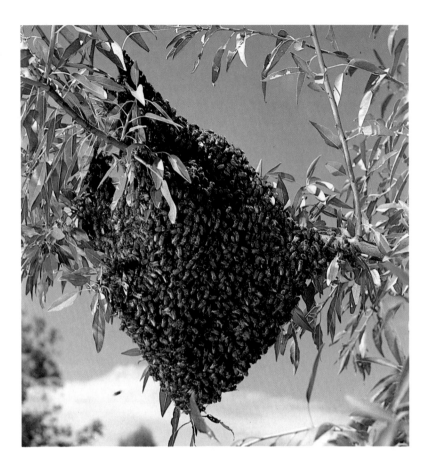

for clustering, foraging, and marking the nest entrance. The results show surprising agreement. In general, the same few components are most important for initiating of all three types of behavior.

One of the critical components of Nasonov pheromone is a compound known as citral, which is also a constituent of the fragrance of oranges. About two years before other investigators identified citral in the Nasonov pheromone, Murray S. Blum foresaw a connection between orange fragrance and honey bee pheromones. Blum is a scientist who has made

significant contributions to several areas of chemical ecology. While walking with his daughters one day, he bought them orange ice cream to eat. A horde of bees soon arrived, clustered about the girls, and pursued them so vigorously that they were forced to throw the ice cream away. Blum noted at the time that the orange flavoring of the ice cream must contain a bee attractant.

Research on the Nasonov pheromone has led to the development of a commercially distributed Nasonov lure. Beekeepers find this synthetic pheromone useful in controlling swarming bees. It also has a market as a bait for traps in food-processing plants, greenhouses, and similar settings where honey bees are undesirable.

Alarm and Aggression Pheromones

In 1609 Charles Butler (who also discovered that drones are male bees) commented in *The Feminine Monarchie, or a Treatise Concerning Bees* that a single bee sting on clothing or skin induces other bees to attack the same site. If a guard bee on duty at the entrance to a hive is disturbed, she opens her sting chamber, protrudes her sting, and releases alarm pheromone. She fans her wings to disseminate her message and runs into the hive to raise the alarm and get help. Excited bees rush out and take up aggressive postures at the entrance.

With jaws wide open, antennae waving, and wings extended, they are ready to fall on the enemy and defend their home.

The alarm pheromone that provokes this swift deployment of defenses comes from cells that are in the sting chamber but not part of the four glands that furnish the sting. The shaft of the sting of a worker bee is barbed and once sunk into vertebrate skin, it cannot be withdrawn. As the bee flies away from its stung victim, the sting and its associated glands separate from the body of the bee and are left behind. This trauma soon kills the bee, but the sting apparatus continues to discharge venom into the victim and alarm pheromone into the surroundings. This marks the site of the initial strike and rallies other bees to the target.

The major component of the alarm pheromone is an ester known as isopentyl acetate. About twenty other constituents have been isolated, and several of them are other similar

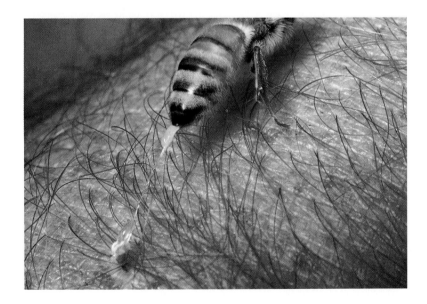

A honey bee after depositing her barbed sting in human skin. As the bee moves away, the sting remains embedded in her victim. The bee is eviscerated and will die, but the sting continues to pump venom into the victim and alarm pheromone into the surroundings.

esters. These are all volatile compounds that are quickly dispersed. Esters of this type have a fruity odor, and in fact isopentyl acetate is a principal component of the odor of bananas. It is not surprising then that angry bees vigorously attack banana oil.

Bioassays for alarm pheromone are difficult to quantitate because the natural response of the bee includes the releasing of more alarm pheromone. Bioassays have shown, however, that several of the esters and alcohols can act alone to alert a colony when presented on a lure at the hive entrance. Isopentyl acetate, for example, both arouses bees and stimulates them to sting. It functions less well, however, than natural alarm pheromone. In a bioassay for stinging behavior, two cotton balls, one treated with the test substance and one a control, are dangled in front of the hive entrance. Stings on each ball are then recorded. Isopentyl acetate plus one other constituent is as satisfactory as the total mixture from natural stings in eliciting the sting response.

Cannibalism Pheromone

Normal drones come from unfertilized eggs laid by the queen. Fertilized eggs routinely develop into workers or new queens. The vagaries of sex determination in the honey bee, however, lead to the occasional development of fertilized eggs into males. Now, workers and queens have a double set of chromosomes, one from their mother and one from their father, just as most organisms do. Individuals having a double set of chromosomes are *diploid*. The normal drones have only half the ordinary complement of chromosomes, because they received chromosomes from their mother but have no father. The aberrant males from fertil-

ized eggs have both a mother and a father and are diploid. The only social contribution drones make is to mate with queens, and diploid males cannot produce offspring. In some other species with a similar genetic mechanism for sex determination, such diploid males simply are not viable, but diploid male honey bees can survive. However, the colony will not tolerate these useless, unproductive extra mouths to feed. Nurse bees typically devour any diploid drone larvae within a few hours of their hatching. Scientists assume that a pheromone brands these abnormal larvae as undesirable, because in experiments nurses consume normal larvae that have been painted with an extract of diploid drone larvae.

A Posthumous Message

Most workers die outside in the course of their labors, but there are still many corpses to clear from within an active hive. For some time after a bee succumbs, workers will continue to approach the body and act as if it is alive. With time, the dead bee begins to decay and liberate oleic acid, a fatty acid we have met before, from its tissues. This substance acts as a pheromone, stimulating workers to move the carcass toward the hive entrance. Removal proceeds in many small steps: passing workers note the signal of oleic acid, pick up the dead bee, and shift it a bit closer to the entrance. Eventually the colony undertakers take over and eject the corpse from the hive. The bee's final, posthumous message has notified its nestmates of its own demise. The signal is apparently irresistible. Workers will pick up and oust a squirming live bee, even a queen, that scientists have painted with oleic acid.

Trail Pheromones and Other Signals Used by Ants

About 8,800 species of ants have been described, and perhaps 20,000 species exist worldwide. Scientists have conducted behavioral and chemical studies of pheromones in several dozen ant species. Both ants and honey bees live communal lives, and several of the messages they employ have similar purposes. Both have alarm pheromones and attractants; both make use of odors to convey information about their brood and its condition. In each, oleic acid from a dead and decomposing nestmate is a signal to dispose of the corpse.

One signal important to ants but not used by honey bees is a trail pheromone. Many ants forage across the countryside in large numbers and undertake mass migrations; these activities proceed because one ant lays a trail on the ground for others to follow. As a worker fire ant returns home after finding a source of food, she marks her route by intermittently touching her sting to the ground and depositing a tiny amount of trail pheromone. These trails incorporate no directional information and may be followed by other fire ants in either direction. E. O. Wilson has written of his discovery of the source of an ant trail pheromone in the late 1950s:

> I was keeping imported fire ants *(Solenopsis invicta)* in culture. The species had always been a favorite of mine since my early work on it in Alabama. Fire ants have a dramatic odor trail system, and so I decided to try to find the source of the chemical scent. Could the key substance come from one of the organs in the posterior region of the abdomen? I painstakingly dissected out the rectal sac and two principal glands of the poison apparatus and washed them individually in insect Ringer's solution—not an easy procedure, since these organs are barely visible to the naked eye. I then crushed each in turn on the tip of an applicator stick and smeared it in an

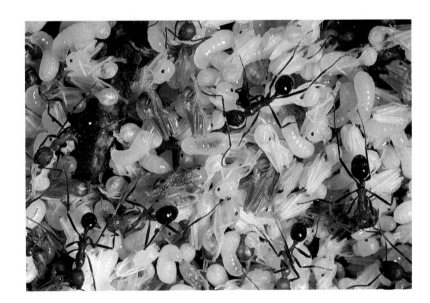

Adult harvester ants with larvae and pupae. Like honey bees and other social insects, ants use a variety of chemical signals in caring for their brood.

artificial trail across the glass plate being used by the fire ants as a foraging arena. At best I expected to find that some of the ants would follow the line when they were later stimulated by the presentation of food. But when I tested Dufour's gland, an insignificant finger-shaped organ located at the base of the sting, an astonishing thing happened. Worker ants poured out of the nest by the dozens, ran the length of the artificial trail, and milled around in confusion at its end.

Several research groups, including that of R. M. Silverstein, have analyzed these trail signals, and we now know chemical constituents of about twenty of them.

Unlike some other messages, such as the one arising from a dead ant, a food trail needs to be kept secret from members of other species. It is not surprising then that ant species use a wide variety of compounds as trail pheromones. Ants can be fantastically sensitive to these signals. Investigators working with the trail pheromone of the leafcutter ant *Atta*

texana calculated that 1 milligram of this substance would suffice to lead a column of ants three times around the earth.

The vapor of the evaporating pheromone over the trail guides an ant along the way, and the ant detects this signal with receptors in its antennae. The illustration shows a set of very pretty experiments carried out by Walter Hangartner at the University of Zurich in his doctoral research. He worked with *Lasius fuliginosus*, an ant that nests in the woods outside Zurich. A trail pheromone will evaporate to furnish the highest concentration of vapor right over the trail, in what we shall call the vapor space. In following a straight trail (*left*), the ant moves to the right and left, oscillating back and forth across the line of the trail itself, bringing first one and then the other antenna into the vapor space. As she moves to the right, her left antenna arrives in the vapor space. The signal it receives causes her to swing to the left, and the ant pursues this new course until her right antenna reaches the vapor space. She then swings back to the right, and so weaves back and forth down the trail. When Hangartner removed the left antenna of the ant (*middle*), she invariably overcorrected to the right. She continues to move to the right, awaiting the signal that the (now absent) left antenna should pick up in the vapor space. Finally she turns back anyway. On her leftward swings, she has no problem, and this portion of her movement is normal. The trail of an ant whose antennae were crossed at the base and glued in this abnormal position with a drop of nail polish is shown (*right*). The ant starts down the trail and promptly becomes confused. She stops frequently to clean her antennae and then progresses, disoriented and evidently bewildered. You might expect that during her mixed-up wanderings, the ant would be just as likely to end up headed back toward her starting point

Trail pheromone of a typical northern European ant, *Myrmica rubra*.

Trail pheromone of the leafcutter ant *Atta texana*.

Trail pheromone of the fire ant *Solenopsis invicta*.

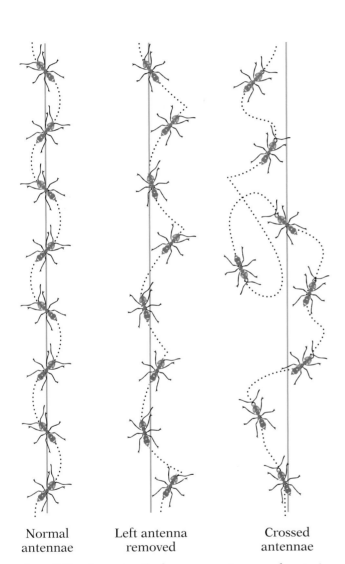

Normal
antennae

Left antenna
removed

Crossed
antennae

Ants following a trail pheromone. A normal ant zig-zags down the trail (*left*). An ant without a left antenna travels too far to the right before turning back to the left (*middle*). An ant with crossed antennae proceeds in confusion (*right*).

as not. In fact, 65 percent of such ants with crossed antennae did slowly make their way to the end of the trail. It took them over five times as long as normal workers to complete the course, but they did not lose their sense of direction. This minor success probably results from nonchemical cues that helped these ants maintain their orientation. For his experiments Hangartner extracted the natural pheromone from other ants of the same species and used this material to lay artificial trails. At the time, he did not know the chemical nature of the signal. Some years later, Max Viscontini and his co-workers at the University of Zurich found that this trail pheromone of *L. fuliginosus* consists of a mixture of simple fatty acids with 6 to 12 carbon atoms.

Ants of some species make slaves of other ants. Scouts belonging to slave-making species lay trails not only to food sources but also to nearby nests of other ants. These scouts return home with a call to battle, and workers pour forth to assault the other colony. The marauding ants follow the scouts' trail to the neighboring nest. They rush in, kill and eat many of the inhabitants, and carry others back to their own nest to live in slavery. One slave-making ant, *Formica subintegra*, has an unusually large gland that holds a reservoir of its alarm pheromone. The signal is a mixture of several esters. Like other alarm pheromones, this blend of esters acts to mobilize *F. subintegra*, but in slave raids it also has another function. The raiding ants use it as an offensive weapon and spray it on their victims. It frightens and disperses the defending ants, creating chaos and confusion in their colony, all to the advantage of the invaders. E. O. Wilson discovered this phenomenon and has called these pheromonal components "propaganda substances." The propaganda substances of at least one species of slave-making ant actually provoke their terrorized victims into fighting one another.

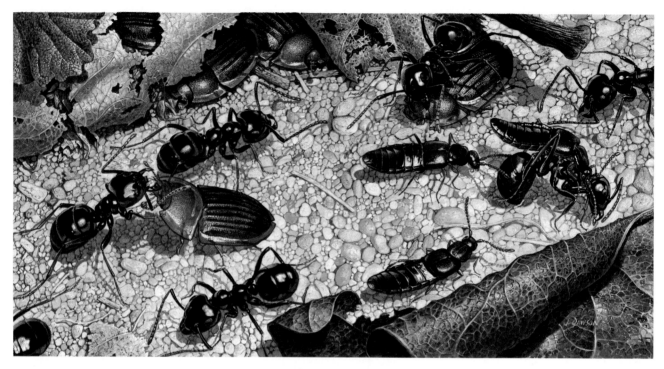

Amphotis marginata beetles along an ant trail. In the foreground a beetle begs food from an ant, while at the rear an ant tries to pry a beetle loose from its protective grasp of the ground. Other *Amphotis* beetles lie in wait beside the trail, and slender *Pella* beetles also hunt for food-laden ants.

Robbery on the Ant Trail

The busy life along ant trails attracts the attention of outsiders. Whereas ants find it advantageous to keep their trails secret from others, other species can turn an ability to follow these trails into a decent livelihood. Ants attract many species that live as their guests or parasites, or as predators on the life of the colony. In certain cases, these outsiders are even more sensitive to the trail pheromones than the ants themselves.

One of the most intriguing of these intruders is *Amphotis marginata*, a beetle that can detect and move along trails of the wood ant *Lasius fuliginosus*, the species that Hangartner used in his experiments on trail following. These ants maintain trails 30 to 60 meters long between their nest and outlying colonies of aphids that they keep and regularly "milk" as an important food source. Ants filled with rich food from the aphids return home along the trails. They are eager to share this nourishment with their nestmates and will regurgitate droplets of food when tapped on the mouth. To take advantage of these ants, the beetle hides in a crack or crevice beside one of the trails. When an ant comes along, the beetle stops her and taps her repeatedly with his antennae. The ant obligingly dispenses a bit of food, and the beetle feeds. Suddenly, the ant seems to recognize that she has been deceived, and she attacks the beetle. The beetle, however, has played this game before and has a nearly perfect defense. It pulls its legs in and uses them to hold itself firmly against the ground, so that only its hard upper surface is exposed. The ant cannot penetrate this shield or turn the beetle over. She soon abandons the effort and continues down the trail. The beetle resumes his post and waits for another ant.

A variety of other species that frequent ants' trails are predators that kill and eat the ants. There are also numerous trail-following beetles that live as guests of army ants. They come along behind raiding parties, reading the trail with no difficulty, and arrive at the site of attack in time to share in the spoils of the ants' battle.

We could easily continue with insect pheromones. The popularity of insects as research subjects and their varied ways offer an almost inexhaustible supply of material. We resist this temptation, however, and instead turn to the attractions of another group. These are the vertebrates, many fewer in number than the insects, but also highly prosperous creatures with a global distribution.

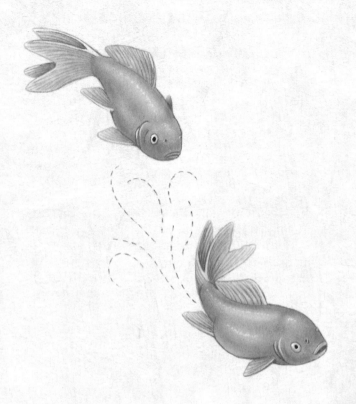
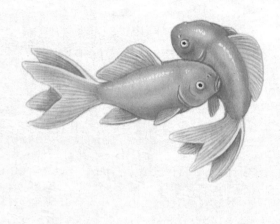
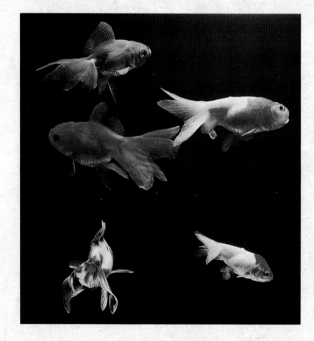

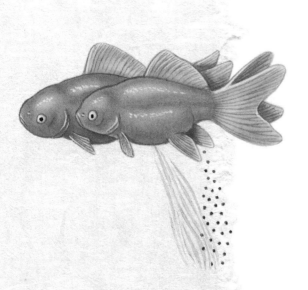

5

SHIFTING FUNCTIONS
AND CHEMICAL
MASQUERADES

■ The hormone that stimulates a female goldfish to release her eggs also acts as a pheromone that signals to males that she is ready to do so. Male goldfish respond by chasing her and pushing her with their heads. Soon, the female discharges her eggs into the water, and one or more males release sperm over them.

*V*ertebrates are familiar from the zoo and aquarium, the farm and the countryside, and perhaps they seem more animal-like than invertebrates. The pheromones of fishes, snakes, and other vertebrate species introduce new considerations and complications. For the first time in our story the distinction between hormones and pheromones breaks down. As we shall see, chemicals that carry messages within one organism also serve as signals to other members of the species. The double function of these chemicals has led scientists to build arguments about the origins of chemical signals. A further complication is that, unlike more simply organized creatures, many vertebrates have two different systems for receiving chemical signals from their environment. Finally, we have an example of pheromone mimicry within a single species: male snakes that have found a reproductive advantage in appearing to be females.

In this chapter we sample pheromones in the vertebrates that are not mammals, saving the mammals for the chapter to follow. In addition to snakes, there are fishes, amphibians, and birds to consider here. We begin with the lamprey, an ancient creature that does not quite qualify as a fish.

Luring Lampreys

The most primitive vertebrates are lampreys and hagfishes. They lack jaws and have a skeleton of cartilage rather than bone. Lampreys

are shaped like eels and are common marine and freshwater predators of fish. They use their round jawless mouths to attach themselves to the body of a fish, which they then assault with rasplike tongues, drawing sustenance from its tissues as prey and predator swim along together.

French fishermen catch lampreys *(Petromyzon marinus)* by placing an adult male in a trap and leaving it overnight in the water. The next day the trap is teeming with females, lured to the male by a potent attractant. Behavioral experiments have demonstrated that the pheromone is in male urine and that males begin to produce the pheromone when they become sexually mature. As in other species, the male's sexual development is under the control of sex hormones. Other studies have established that testosterone, the common steroidal male sex hormone, is present in the urine of male lampreys, and that its concentration increases sharply at sexual maturity. Could testosterone be the pheromone?

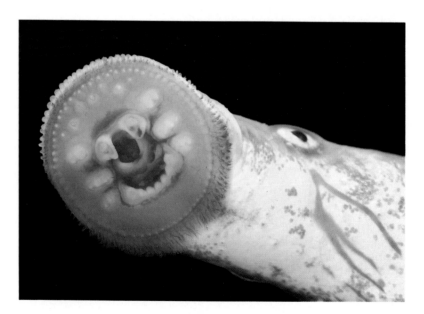

A lamprey attaches itself to its prey by this rounded oral disc, or mouth cup. The toothed tongue in the center is an effective substitute for jaws in rasping off the flesh of the lamprey's prey.

In a bioassay, testosterone acts as an attractant for female lampreys at the low concentration of 29 picograms per milliliter. The bioassay is set up so that a female lamprey can choose between two compartments in a test tank. The substance being assayed is added to the water in one compartment, and the other compartment serves as a control. The female has free access to each compartment, and the time she spends in each of them over a fixed period is recorded. Her preference for the sample is scored as excess time in the test compartment. Although isolated testosterone is highly attractive, male urine is even more attractive. Urine continues to attract females in this bioassay even when the final diluted concentration of testosterone present is only one ten-thousandth (1×10^{-4}) as great as the lowest attractive concentration of pure testosterone. The attractivity of urine is obviously much too great to be explained solely by the presence of testosterone. There must be at least one additional component that either is

Testosterone

very effective itself or else greatly enhances the attractivity of testosterone. So far no one knows what this substance might be.

The presence of sex attractants in urine appears to be a common phenomenon in fishes. There is evidence in at least three different species of bony fishes, which include most of the species that we think of as fishes, that steroidal sex hormones in male urine serve as female attractants. Analysis shows the steroids are present in the urine, and in behavioral experiments such compounds are active attractants. In no case, however, is the story

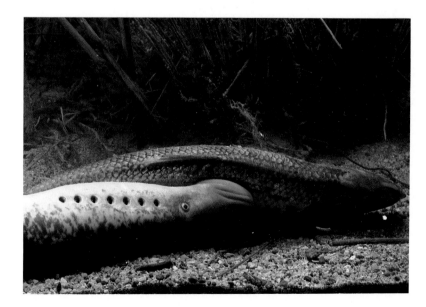

A lamprey and its prey. As they swim, the lamprey takes its nourishment directly from the victim's body.

yet complete. It may be that, as in the lamprey, more than one component is required to provide the full pheromonal activity of urine. Such an arrangement could possibly enhance the specificity of attraction. One active component common to many species might be testosterone, and then additional components could create a signal attractive to only a single species. Such an arrangement would have an obvious advantage, for without it a variety of species might respond to a single signal. Wooing only legitimate potential mates would be more efficient than soliciting the advances of a random mix of neighbors. We shall have more to say shortly about the concept of a hormone such as testosterone also serving as a pheromone.

Fishes

The fishes are the most abundant and diverse of the vertebrates, and apart from lampreys and hagfishes their evolutionary lineage dates back the farthest. Most fishes have a bony skeleton and are grouped together as "bony fishes." Over their long history, these creatures have evolved a wide variety of reproductive modes and behaviors. Some fishes build nests and care for their young; some practice pair bonding; some are utterly promiscuous. Their methods of fertilization vary and so do their approaches to care for fertilized eggs. Opportunities abound for pheromones, and in fact, there are reports that chemical signals regulate a host of reproductive activities in fishes, including parent-young interactions, homing, attracting a mate, pair formation, sexual recognition, and spawning. In addition to reproductive pheromones, there is evidence for signals associated with schooling and avoiding enemies. In most cases this research is just at its beginning, and details of the biology and

chemistry of these pheromones have not yet been explored.

A set of pretty behavioral observations of this sort from the 1930s concerns pair formation in the blind goby *Typhlogobius californiensis*. This is a bright pink, intertidal fish, about 6 centimeters (2.5 inches) long. Pairs of gobies live in the deepest parts of gravelly burrows constructed by the ghost shrimp *Callianassa affinis*. Although newly hatched blind gobies have perfectly developed eyes, after they take up residence in a shrimp burrow, their eyes degenerate and disappear. Gobies pair for life, which is up to twelve years, with pairs forming before they are six months old. Typically a pair remains in one burrow throughout their lifetimes, leaving only if forcibly evicted.

Pair formation is simply a matter of sexual recognition plus the fact that a goby will only tolerate other gobies of the opposite sex. The blind goby at the bottom of the shrimp burrow is able to distinguish between male and female gobies. If a third blind goby is introduced into a burrow occupied by a pair of gobies, the resident goby of the same sex attacks it. These fish are extremely aggressive, and the battle between the two fish continues until one of them is either killed or driven from the burrow. If the newcomer is the victor, the surviving original resident accepts its new mate with no indication that it is aware of any change. Pair formation does not include individual recognition but is merely the result of each goby's acceptance only of the opposite sex.

A simple experiment demonstrated that a chemical signal mediates the blind goby's sexual and species recognition, and this provided one of the earliest indications that fishes use pheromones. An investigator inserted a male blind goby in a sealed bag of water into the burrow of a pair of gobies. The residents ignored this intrusion until the investigator

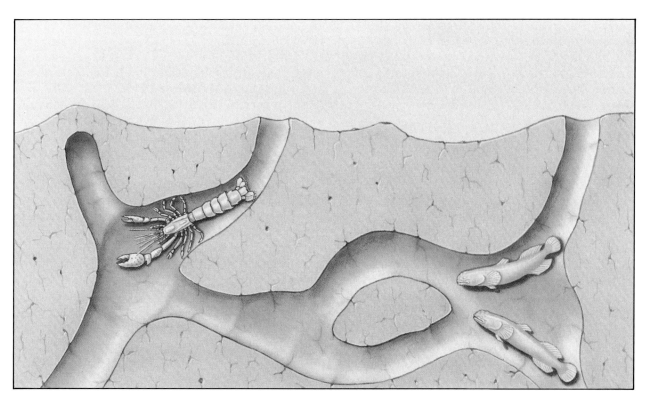

A pair of blind gobies living in the burrow dug in sandy mud by a ghost shrimp.

punctured the bag and the water inside began to flow out. As soon as water from the bag reached the resident male, he began to attack the bag fiercely. Presumably the water from the bag carried with it a chemical signal emitted by the new fish that marked it as a male blind goby.

There are many other examples of chemical communication in fishes that have been explored less thoroughly than this signal in the goby. However, two pheromonal systems have been studied in detail and deserve our extended consideration.

Fright Reactions from an Alarm Substance

The vast majority of the world's river and lake fishes belong to a group of bony fishes called ostariophysians, which comprises more than 5000 species. Most of the familiar freshwater species are here: carp, catfish, and goldfish. This group includes many species of minnows, and one of these, the European minnow *Phoxinus phoxinus,* has been an important subject of pheromone research. We described in

Chapter 1 Karl von Frisch's discovery of the fright reaction in *P. phoxinus* and noted that an alarm substance contained in skin cells of the fish is responsible for this behavior.

While the fright reaction is common to most ostariophysians, there are some species that have alarm-system cells but do not show the reaction. The cells of these species are fully loaded with the signal, and extracts of their skin will elicit fright in responsive species. This observation has led some scientists to conclude that the alarm substance originally had a different function. Perhaps it was a toxin to discourage predators, for example. According to this suggestion, the ostariophysians later evolved responsiveness that enabled them to use the substance as a pheromone. There are also a few of these fishes that have neither the cells nor the reaction. In the majority that do react, the alarm substance from one species generally seems to produce the reaction in others.

Fifty years of investigation has yielded a large body of information about behavioral and physiological aspects of the ostariophysian fright reaction. A fish becomes visually more alert and its heartbeat slows as part of the reaction. Ostariophysians that do not show overt fright do show these same physiological changes. We also know that a compound called hypoxanthine-3-oxide (H3O) is the major component of the pheromone. Max Viscontini and his student M. Argentini, chemists at the University of Zurich, have collaborated with biologist Wolfgang Pfeiffer and his research group at the University of Tübingen on this problem.

These investigators extracted the skin of *P. phoxinus* and then removed proteins from the extract to obtain a crude active concen-

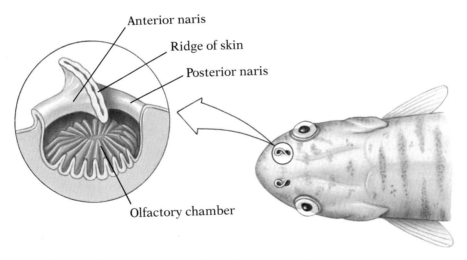

The European minnow detects alarm pheromone through its sense of smell. As the minnow swims, a ridge of skin on each side of its head directs water through an opening known as the anterior naris and into the olfactory chamber. After passing over the olfactory cells, the water leaves through the posterior naris.

H3O

trate. From this they prepared a purified fraction that was quite active in provoking the fright reaction and that they identified as H3O. They then showed that pure H3O prepared in the laboratory is also highly active. H3O is somewhat unstable in water and decomposes slowly to other substances that have no pheromonal activity. This is an appropriate property for the pheromone, since it is undesirable for an alarm signal to accumulate in the environment.

The investigators do not know yet whether H3O is as active as the natural pheromone. To make this comparison they need to quantify the fright reaction. We have seen how a bioassay can measure attractivity semiquantitatively, but how can a scientist quantify fright? Pfeiffer and his students have devised a test for the pheromone that may answer this question. Their bioassay is based on the observation that in the presence of the alarm substance, but not at other times, a small freshwater fish, the black tetra *Gymnocorymbus ternetzi*, reacts to a source of light by turning its body in a predictable and reproducible manner. Interestingly, this response is accompanied by measurable changes in the central nervous system of the fish. If Pfeiffer finds that these physiological changes reflect in a simple way the amount of alarm substance being tested, this ingenious bioassay may furnish the desired quantitative measure of the fright reaction in the near future.

Stimulating Production of Milt

There is quite a bit of evidence that various events in the reproduction of fishes are under pheromonal control. We have noted that pheromones of several animals appear to be steroidal sex hormones or compounds closely related to them. The behaviorally and chemically most complete investigations of steroidal pheromones pertain to the goldfish *Carassius auratus*. Two different signals from the female goldfish control the reproductive physiology and behavior of the male. Owing to wideranging studies initiated by Norman E. Stacey at the University of Alberta, we have an unusually complete picture of the mode of action of these two pheromones. This research on goldfish reproductive signals provides perhaps the best illustration of how chemical signals are physiologically integrated into a vertebrate organism.

To make these investigations meaningful, we must first say a bit about reproduction in the goldfish. These familiar fishes do not build nests or care for their young. After ovulation, the females holds her eggs within her body for several hours. Postovulatory females are said to be ripe, meaning they are ready to release their eggs, or spawn. A ripe female spawns in the midst of a group of goldfish, with several males chasing, nudging, and competing for her. In natural habitats the female eventually permits herself to be pushed in among aquatic plants, where she releases her eggs in synchrony with discharge of milt (sperm and seminal fluid) by one or more of the attendant males. Fertilization takes place in the water, and then the eggs scatter over the nearby plants. The adult fishes pay no further attention to either eggs or progeny.

Like other fishes that abandon their fertilized eggs or young, goldfish discharge great

One of the many fancy varieties of goldfish, the red lionhead veiltail.

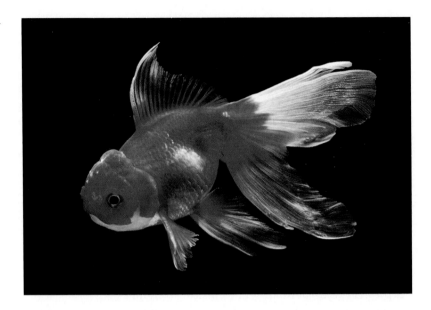

numbers of eggs at each spawning. Commercial breeders can strip eggs or milt manually
from a goldfish by applying slight pressure to
the abdomen while holding the fish. The
breeders thoroughly mix expelled eggs and
milt in a container and then pour the mixture
into an aquarium. Ten thousand eggs from a
single female can be inseminated at a time in
this fashion.

Stacey and his collaborators discovered
that the two reproductive pheromones sent
from female goldfish to males also act as hormones that carry chemical signals within the
female. In the hours before ovulation, the concentration of a certain steroidal sex hormone
increases in the blood of the female. This hormone, which we can call 17,20P, stimulates
final maturation of the female's eggs. As the
concentration of 17,20P builds up, the female
begins to discharge the hormone, which diffuses through the water and reaches male
goldfish. 17,20P now acts as a pheromone,

causing a dramatic increase in the male's accumulation of milt over the next 8 to 10
hours. Males exposed overnight to low concentrations of 17,20P yield over five times as
much milt as males that do not receive the
pheromone. This signal sent by the ripe female
improves her chances of having her eggs fertilized at spawning and improves the male's
chances of passing on his genes. Because many
males may discharge milt near one spawning

17,20P

female, the volume of milt a male discharges is probably a significant factor in his reproductive success.

Interestingly, Stacey's discovery of the pheromonal action of 17,20P was an accident. He and a colleague had injected 17,20P into male goldfish to study its effect on milt production. They were surprised to find that control males held in the same tank also produced more milt, even though these controls had received no injections of 17,20P. The investigators eventually discovered that a minute concentration of 17,20P, presumably released into the tank water by the injected males, induced this response by the controls.

Stacey and his collaborators have examined how the 17,20P signal causes an increase in milt volume. They found that the male detects the pheromone when the water contains only a tiny fraction of a picogram per milliliter, demonstrating an extraordinarily high sensitivity to this steroid. About 3 grams of 17,20P (about a teaspoonful) would provide this threshold concentration throughout the water in a tank that was a cube 500 meters on a side! Stacey and his colleagues found that this sensitive detection takes place through the olfactory system of the male goldfish, and this was the first evidence that the olfactory system of a fish could detect such a low concentration of a chemical compound. Scientists often simply assume that olfaction is the pathway for detection of a pheromone, but here there is a set of experiments that establishes the point nicely. Surgical interruption of the male olfactory system completely inhibits the effects of 17,20P on the male, clearly establishing the mode of detection. On detecting the pheromone, the olfactory system passes a signal to the brain. The brain processes the signal by a series of steps that are not yet worked out for this or any other pheromone.

We do know, however, that as a consequence of the brain's processing, the signal is sent to the pituitary gland. This gland, located at the base of the brain, is the agent through which the vertebrate brain exercises control over the gonads. The pituitary accomplishes this by manufacturing protein hormones and releasing them into the blood. The hormones travel around the body in the circulation and are detected by receptors in the gonads, which then respond appropriately to the specific hormone and its message.

In the male goldfish a pituitary hormone known as gonadotropin regulates the functioning of the testes. The signal from the brain to the pituitary elicits secretion of gonadotropin into the blood, and the elevated concentration of gonadotropin stimulates the testes to greater milt formation. As you would expect, the level of gonadotropin in the blood of male goldfish does indeed rise after he is exposed to 17,20P. Scientists also studied males whose pituitary glands had been surgically removed and found that 17,20P has no effect on milt volume in these fish. This investigation confirmed that milt production increases because of the chain of events just discussed.

The level of detailed understanding of 17,20P in goldfish is probably unique among studies of single pheromones in vertebrates. In this one case we know the chemical structure of the pheromone, its source, and details of its release by the female. In the recipient male we know the sensory pathway for detection, the physiological changes it induces, the observable result of these changes, and the consequences of this result for both sender and receiver of the signal. For many pheromones some details analogous to these are known and others can be guessed at. For 17,20P in goldfish, we have experimental evidence for the entire sequence of events.

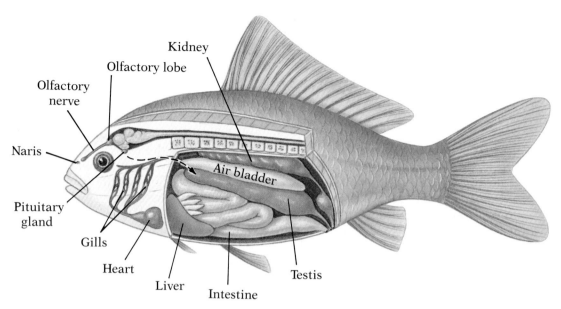

The major organs of a male goldfish, including those (in purple) that have a role in the action of the pheromone 17,20P emitted by the female. Once the pheromone has been detected by the olfactory system, a signal travels through the nervous system to the pituitary gland, which then sends a hormone through the bloodstream to the testes.

Getting Eggs and Milt Together

17,20P readied the male for reproduction by triggering an increased accumulation of milt. Now a second signal attracts males to the female just as she ovulates. Male fish appear to recognize that the female is ready to spawn: they begin to chase her, butt her with their heads, and investigate the sides of her body with their snouts. Stacey investigated this attractant pheromone as well and found that one of its components is a prostaglandin that also acts as a female hormone.

In discussing the hatching pheromone of the arctic barnacle, we mentioned that prostaglandins are found in many vertebrates and invertebrates, and we spoke of the importance of prostaglandins in human biology and medicine. In female goldfish the concentrations of two prostaglandins, called $PGF_{2\alpha}$ and 15-keto-$PGF_{2\alpha}$, increase at the time of ovulation. $PGF_{2\alpha}$ is a hormone that acts directly on the female's

Prostaglandin $F_{2\alpha}$ ($PGF_{2\alpha}$)

brain in connection with spawning, and 15-keto-PGF$_{2\alpha}$ is a closely related compound. Stacey suspected that these two PGFs were also the pheromone that attracted males to the female. He discovered that they were present in the water at the right time to act as an attractant, because the female discharges them rapidly after PGF$_{2\alpha}$ has delivered its hormonal message. When he injected these PGFs into female goldfish, the fish exhibited spawning behavior and became attractive to males. Stacey's collaborators next determined that males are indeed very sensitive to these compounds. They found that male olfactory receptor cells (cells that are the primary detectors of odorants) respond to PGF$_{2\alpha}$ at the very low concentration of 35 picograms per milliter and that these cells are a hundred times more sensitive to 15-keto-PGF$_{2\alpha}$.

These scientists then demonstrated that the male's reaction to the PGFs is the same as to the natural pheromone. In the critical behavioral bioassay, they found that appropriately low concentrations of the PGFs provoked spawning behavior in male fish. The males began to chase and nudge, just as they did in

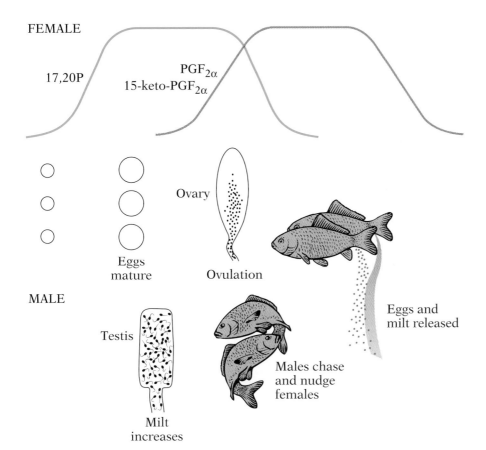

FEMALE

17,20P

PGF$_{2\alpha}$
15-keto-PGF$_{2\alpha}$

Ovary

Eggs mature

Ovulation

Eggs and milt released

Males chase and nudge females

MALE

Testis

Milt increases

The two reproductive pheromones of the female goldfish coordinate mating events. The amounts of these pheromones released rise and fall over time, stimulating the development and release of eggs and eliciting a sequence of responses in the male.

the presence of a ripe female. Collectively, these experiments proved that the two PGFs released by the female after ovulation act as an attractant pheromone for male goldfish.

We now see that the female goldfish discharges two compounds, 17,20P and $PGF_{2\alpha}$, after they have served their purpose as reproductive hormones, along with a third compound, 15-keto-$PGF_{2\alpha}$. After being released into the water, these compounds act as pheromones for the male goldfish. Together these signals coordinate male and female reproductive physiology and spawning behavior. We saw earlier that the sex hormone testosterone is a female attractant in the sea lamprey. In three instances, one compound serves as both hormone and pheromone. When Peter Karlson and Martin Lüscher coined the word *pheromone* to designate chemical signals passed among members of a single species, they intentionally made a distinction between pheromones and hormones. One was discharged externally into the environment, and the other secreted internally within an organism. We now find that this distinction can break down.

Pheromones from Hormones and Vice Versa

Chemical signals are primitive and widespread. We noted early on that in many organisms they are the primary mode of communication within a species. Some scientists have argued that hormones turned into pheromones, that is, that chemicals already in use as internal signals were adapted for communication between individuals. Other investigators have made the converse argument: external signals already in use between early unicellular organisms were transformed into internal

signals as simple organisms evolved into multicellular species, and pheromones thus became hormones.

The two arguments need not be mutually exclusive; both can be true. It seems very probable that in particular instances chemicals have changed their function in each of the two directions postulated. Steroids and prostaglandins exist throughout the animal kingdom and have well-recognized hormonal functions. With this in mind, it seems natural to regard the employment of 17,20P and $PGF_{2\alpha}$ as pheromones in the goldfish as adaptations using pre-existing hormones. In the simplest version of this course of events, these compounds would be discharged into the water at the appropriate times as a consequence of their use as hormones. Over evolutionary time, sensitive receptors for these compounds and suitable physiological or behavioral responses to them would gradually evolve in the male and the excreted hormones would thereby acquire an auxiliary role as pheromones. We could similarly explain how the testosterone in male lamprey's urine came to be an attractant for the female.

This argument can be extended to pheromones that appear to have been originally present in the environment not as hormones, but for some other reason. Recall that larval arctic barnacles prefer to settle on surfaces already colonized by their own species and that this behavior reflects their attraction to the protein arthropodin. The protein slowly leaches from the cuticle of sessile adult barnacles into the surrounding water. It seems likely that the protein was there, passively dissolving from the cuticle and diffusing away into the environment, and that larval barnacles subsequently evolved a response to the protein. We saw a related situation in the dog tick. Cholesteryl oleate on the surface of the female dog tick appears to have undergone transformation from a simple waste product to a pheromone.

Amphibians

The main living amphibians are frogs, toads, and salamanders. Their forbears made the momentous evolutionary advance to life on the land, although these creatures have never made a complete break with the water. Their eggs must remain wet, or at least damp, to survive. Even tree frogs that never descend to the ground deposit their eggs in the moist crannies and forks of their trees, and some other amphibians keep their eggs moist in more esoteric ways, such as those frogs that carry their eggs in their mouths until they hatch. Still other amphibians lead lives quite closely tied to water. As a consequence, the penetration of this group in the modern world is limited.

Very little is known about pheromones among these creatures. One exception is an efficient alarm pheromone used by tadpoles of the common toad *Bufo bufo*. When an injured tadpole is introduced into a group, a fright reaction takes place similar to the one in *Phoxinus* and other freshwater fishes. This observation inspired the screening of many other frogs and toads for a similar effect, but with little success. The pheromone is apparently confined to *B. bufo* and its close relatives. In general, frogs and toads use their vocal abilities to attract mates, and their skins lack glands that could produce pheromones.

Salamanders are a more likely source of chemical signals. They generate numerous secretions from glands in their moist skin, on the head, and elsewhere. Some of these secretions are poisons and effective repellents of predators, but others seem to mediate individ-

ual, species, and sex recognition. There has been very little attention to the chemical nature of these glandular secretions, and what little information there is about pheromones in salamanders comes from behavioral observations. One of the best-investigated topics here is courtship, where there is substantial evidence that chemical signals released by the male are important. Most likely these signals foster receptivity in the female during the sometimes intricate interactions of salamander courtship.

Some salamanders also show territorial behavior, which means that they stake out a specific territory, advertise it as their own, and defend it against encroachment. A territorial salamander fights other members of its species when they intrude and typically succeeds in ousting the intruder. One way of laying claim to a particular domain is to mark it with a pheromone. There is behavioral evidence that salamanders do use pheromones to establish their territories, but little is yet known about the biology or chemistry of these chemical signals.

The Vomeronasal Organ

In the course of evolution the reptiles were the first vertebrates to free themselves fully from life in the water. Their achievement brought them great success, and for ages they were the dominant species throughout the globe. Even if reptiles no longer rule the earth, turtles, snakes and lizards, and alligators and crocodiles remain well known, widespread, successful creatues in our world. Pheromones in these animals have received little attention, although there were scattered inquiries as long ago as the 1930s. Vision is generally regarded as the best-developed sense in reptiles, but

With its tongue extended, a common European grass snake *Natrix natrix* samples molecules in the environment.

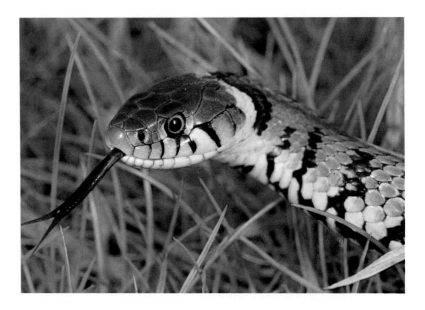

chemical signals are doubtless more consequential than our current knowledge reflects. There is some evidence for chemical communication in lizards and turtles, and considerably more in snakes. Most often, detailed biological and chemical studies are lacking.

The only available information about pheromones of certain snakes and lizards is reports of the rate of tongue flicking in a variety of environmental situations. Anyone who has watched a snake is aware of the frequent flicking of its tongue by which it samples the air and nearby objects. In snakes and some lizards tongue flicking is part of an essential pathway for receiving chemical signals. Chemicals are picked up by the tongue and detected in a sensory organ prominent in many reptiles and mammals but not found in other vertebrates or in invertebrates. This is the vomeronasal organ. Animals that have a vomeronasal

organ depend on it for the detection of many pheromonal signals.

The vomeronasal organ is important in snakes, some lizards, and nonprimate mammals. There is good fossil evidence that it was well developed in now-extinct early lizards and therapsids, which were mammal-like reptiles. In some primates, including man, it makes a transitory appearance during embryological development but disappears before birth. It was first described in 1811 by L. Jacobson, a Danish physician, and is sometimes still referred to as Jacobson's organ. The function and significance of this structure have become clearer in the past ten to fifteen years, but there remains much to learn about its operation. Anatomists and physiologists began to confirm that the role of the vomeronasal organ is to detect chemical signals at roughly the same time that studies of chemical communication suggested there must be some means of detecting chemical signals in addition to the primary olfactory system.

The vomeronasal organ is very similar in structure to the primary olfactory system, but it provides an alternative pathway to the brain. Nerve impulses from the olfactory sensory cells pass to parts of the brain known as the olfactory bulbs. Nerve impulses from sensory cells of the vomeronasal organ enter separate brain structures known as the accessory olfactory bulbs and also project to brain structures that regulate sexual behavior and the secretion of gonadotropin. The vomeronasal organ itself is typically situated in a pouch off the nasal cavity. Airborne odorant molecules reach the olfactory receptor cells as air passes through the nasal cavity, but they cannot efficiently enter the dead-end passage containing the vomeronasal organ in this fashion.

The vomeronasal organ requires another delivery system. In snakes, molecules enter the vomeronasal organ through ducts that connect it with the oral cavity. During flicking, the tongue picks up molecules from the air and nearby objects. As the tongue retracts into the mouth at the end of each flick, the tips of the tongue slide past the openings of these connecting ducts. This moves molecules collected in the environment from the tongue into the ducts and up into the vomeronasal organ, where they reach its receptor cells and are detected.

Mammals have evolved a different delivery system. When they lick and sniff, molecules from the environment are absorbed onto the nose and tongue. These molecules are then transported into the vomeronasal organ in saliva. The organ in mammals is typically cigar-shaped and open at only one end. A pumping action that dilates and constricts the organ walls increases the motion of fluid in and out, and molecules from the environment are moved rapidly into the chamber.

Many animals that have this accessory olfactory system use it to detect chemical sig-

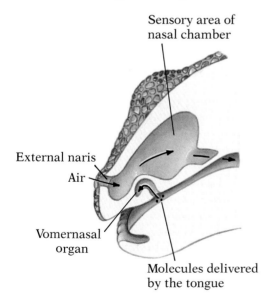

Sensory area of
nasal chamber

External naris

Air

Vomernasal
organ

Molecules delivered
by the tongue

The olfactory apparatus of a lizard. The primary olfactory system in the nasal chamber detects molecules borne on air from the environment, and the accessory olfactory system in the vomeronasal organ detects molecules brought into the mouth on the tongue.

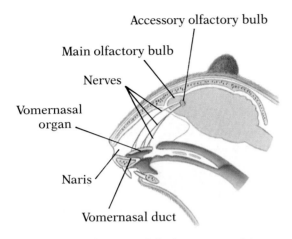

Accessory olfactory bulb

Main olfactory bulb

Nerves

Vomernasal organ

Naris

Vomernasal duct

The vomeronasal organ of the hamster and its neural connections to the accessory olfactory bulb in the brain. Other nerves (not shown) connect the primary olfactory cells in the nasal cavity with the main olfactory bulb.

nals associated with sexual behavior, aggressive responses, and interactions between mother and young. In many species the accessory olfactory system is not an optional second pathway, but rather the required mode of detection for particular pheromonal messages. The next example illustrates its essential role in the sexual behavior of a common snake.

The Mating Pheromone of the Red-Sided Garter Snake

The red-sided garter snake *Thamnophis sirtalis parietalis* has a pheromone that permits males to recognize females. Research on this signal is unusually thorough and interesting in itself, and it has also led to a pheromone that identifies males and to the discovery of a striking example of pheromonal mimicry in these snakes. The original observations concerning

this mating pheromone go back more than fifty years, but we owe much of this remarkable story to laboratory and field research carried out over the past decade at the University of Texas under the leadership of David Crews. Crews is a behavioral biologist whose enthusiasm for snakes appeared early. As a child, he brought snakes home so often that before washing his clothes his mother turned out his pockets with a pencil, checking for specimens.

The red-sided garter snake has a broad range that extends farther north than that of any other reptile in North America. It spends the bitter winters of the northern Great Plains and the Canadian prairies hibernating in large communal dens, each holding up to ten thousand snakes. In the spring the males all emerge more or less at the same time and gather in large groups near the dens. Their aggregates can number into the thousands. They are waiting for females, which appear singly or in small groups over the next several weeks. When a female emerges from her den, she is approached by a band of males, perhaps ten to twenty, but often up to a hundred. In the courtship that follows, these males and the female form a "mating ball," a writhing mass of dozens of 60-centimeter-long (2-foot-long) snakes.

Courtship begins when a male recognizes a female through a pheromone on her back. The pheromone is not volatile. Rapid flicks of the male's tongue transfer the pheromone from the female to his vomeronasal organ. Males whose tongues have been removed do not engage in courtship behavior. In the confusion of a mating ball there may be an advantage in the identifying pheromone being closely associated with the body of the female. After identifying the female, a courting male presses his chin along her back and moves rapidly back and forth along the entire length of her body.

This "chin rubbing," as it is called, is an essential component of the sexual behavior of these snakes, and they do not exhibit it at other times.

Eventually the successful courting male comes to rest with his body and the female's aligned side by side in the same direction and positioned for copulation. Needless to say, this is not a smooth, straightforward undertaking if fifty or a hundred other, less successful males are struggling to do exactly the same thing at the same time. Copulation lasts about 15 minutes, and during this time the unsuccessful males disperse to await another female. Only one male wins the female, and she mates only once each year. She is not receptive to further attention once she has mated, and the successful male leaves behind a pheromone that renders her unattractive to future suitors. These tumultuous events all take place within the first half-hour after the female emerges from hibernation. Females of *T. s. parietalis* ovulate

six or eight weeks after mating, or even later, and the eggs are then fertilized. During this time, the sperm received at mating move slowly to the site of fertilization within the female's body.

Recall that the pheromone exciting the male to courtship is on the back of the female until the male picks it up with his tongue. This observation was puzzling for some years, because the skin of the red-sided garter snake lacks glands that might produce, conserve, or secrete any chemical signal. Scientists finally determined that the pheromone is carried in the bloodstream from where it is produced within the female's body to the deeper layers of her skin, which is porous and thin enough in certain critical areas that substances can diffuse through it onto the surface of the back.

For the attempts to isolate the pheromone that followed these discoveries, male courtship behavior provided a practical bioassay. Because males engage in chin rubbing only in

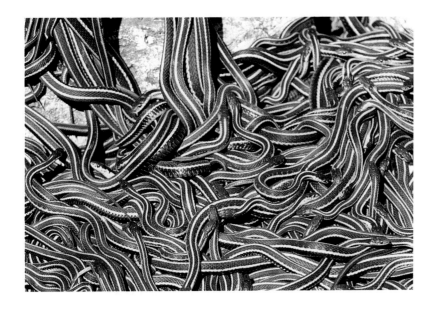

A mass of red-sided garter snakes.

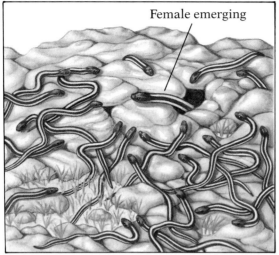

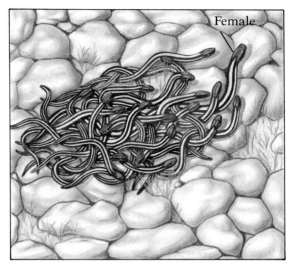

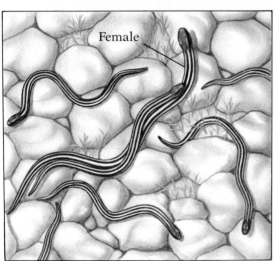

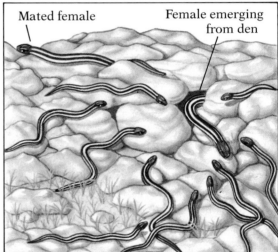

Mating behavior of the red-sided garter snake. *Upper left:* Male snakes
emerge from hibernation and sun themselves near their den, waiting
for the more slowly emerging females. *Upper right:* Soon after a female
appears, they are attracted by the pheromone on her back and form a
mating ball about her. *Lower left:* One male finally succeeds in align-
ing himself along the female's body and then in mating with her. The
unsuccessful males depart to seek another female. *Lower right:* The
mated female, marked with a pheromone by her mating partner, is no
longer attractive to male snakes, and she immediately leaves the vicinity of the den. Males remain near the den, awaiting the emergence
of another unmated female.

response to the pheromone, test fractions could be evaluated by applying them to the back of a male snake and then scoring the incidence of chin rubbing. Skin from attractive females was extracted, and these extracts were then separated into fractions containing proteins, lipids (fats), and other constituents. Extracts containing skin proteins were inactive, but fractions rich in lipids elicited enthusiastic chin rubbing.

By this time the blood had been recognized as the source of the pheromone isolated from skin. Because the male snakes had responded to lipid-rich fractions in the bioassays, scientists decided to study the lipids circulating in the blood of females. They analyzed the blood lipids of receptive and unreceptive female snakes and found a conspicuous difference. The blood of receptive females carried a well-known protein called vitellogenin that is found in many species. This protein is synthesized in the liver and sent to the ovaries as a raw material for yolk formation. Vitellogenin (the Latin *vitellus* means *yolk*) consists of about 1,700 amino acid units. This protein turned up in the investigation of lipids because it has lipid and carbohydrate (sugar) groups attached to some of the amino acids as part of its structure. Of course, once investigators found vitellogenin in receptive females, it was important to test its pheromonal activity. Purified vitellogenin applied to the backs of male snakes elicited courtship behavior in test males, but only if the vitellogenin came from the red-sided garter snake. Samples of the vitellogenin extracted from other species of garter snake, or from a lizard or a chick, had no effect on male red-sided garter snakes.

Up to this point, the results pointed to vitellogenin itself as the mating pheromone, but further experiments cast doubt on this idea. Several bits of information were suggestive, but one fact was convincing. While it was certain that vitellogenin is present deep in the skin, the protein could not be found on the skin's outer surface, where the pheromone had to be. Vitellogenin itself was not the pheromone, but it had pheromonal activity and was somehow essential to the appearance of the pheromone on the female's back.

As Crews reasoned next, if vitellogenin itself is not the pheromone, some lipid that it brings to the skin, and that is then secreted to the surface, must be the active signal. The next experiments had to be the fractionation and identification of the chemical compounds making up the lipids found in the skin of these snakes. Crews, together with investigators at the laboratories of the National Institutes of Health in Bethesda, Maryland, isolated and analyzed lipids from the skin of both males and receptive females. The females yielded much more lipid than the males, an average of 38 milligrams each, versus 8 milligrams from the males. The total lipid extract from the males did not promote chin rubbing in the bioassay, but the total lipid extract from the females did. Purification separated the lipids from the females into 21 fractions, only one of which was active. This active material was discovered to be a mixture of compounds having a long chain in the range of 29 to 37 carbon atoms and containing a carbonyl group. Some of the compounds also contained a double bond. A typical component having 31 carbon atoms and a double bond is illustrated.

A typical component of the mating pheromone of the red-sided garter snake. Some components have no double bond. Those that do have a double bond all have the Z configuration.

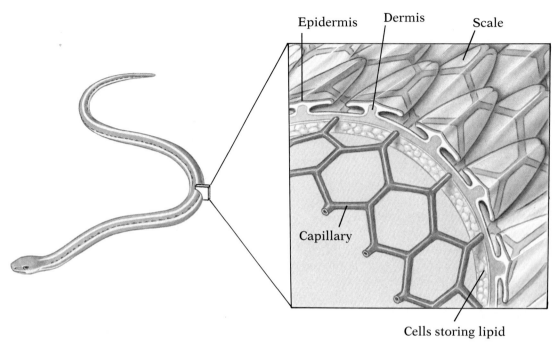

Epidermis   Dermis   Scale

Capillary

Cells storing lipid

The female red-sided garter snake's attractant pheromone moves from the blood, up through the skin (dermis and epidermis), and onto her back. The pheromone passes readily through a thin area of skin between the scales (the hinge region).

The individual components of this mixture were tested in bioassays. The compounds without a double bond were attractive to males, but those carrying the double bond were much more attractive and indeed not significantly different from the natural pheromone. If this mixture of compounds is the pheromone that is secreted onto the backs of receptive female snakes, what is the role of vitellogenin? It seems likely that vitellogenin functions simply as a carrier for the pheromone. Presumably the lipid portion of vitellogenin transports the pheromone in some form and delivers it to the lower layers of the skin. The pheromone could be released there from the vitellogenin lipids and secreted to the surface. While this is a reasonable hypothesis, this aspect of the story still needs experimental attention.

Crews and his collaborators also found lipids in the skin of males, and this permitted another question to be settled. In the wild, male red-sided garter snakes investigate all members of their species during the mating period. After cursory inspection they ignore most other males, but begin exuberant courtship with receptive females. How do the courting males tell male from female? Two possible explanations come to mind. One possibility is that males lack the attractive pheromone of the female that we have just described. Alternatively, they carry some other signal that advertises their maleness, something that we can call a male-recognition pheromone.

Studies of the lipids obtained from male skin support the second explanation. These lipids do contain the compounds found in the female mating pheromone, although in somewhat altered proportions. They also contain something else. When the total male lipids were added to active female extracts, males no longer responded to these extracts in the bioassay. Some component of the male lipid extract must inhibit a positive reaction to the female mating pheromone. Chemical analysis of the male lipids revealed a component not found in the females, and this was identified as the common and widely distributed hydrocarbon squalene. Addition of squalene to the active female pheromone reduced the courtship response of males, but pure squalene was less effective than the complete lipid extract of male skin. It appears then that squalene is one constituent of this male-recognition pheromone and that other active components remain to be identified.

Although the relationship of vitellogenin to the female mating pheromone has not yet been worked out in detail, we do know that the protein has an important overall effect on mating. This effect depends on the amount of vitellogenin present in the female, and it comes about in an interesting way. You will recall that courtship and mating take place as soon as the female appears from hibernation, and that ovulation and fertilization take place several weeks later. After a long winter in the den, a number of the female's physiological functions are at a low point, and this includes the functioning of the ovaries. It is only after mating that the ovaries become fully operative and the development of eggs gets under way. Another consequence of hibernation is that no vitellogenin is being synthesized in the liver at the time of mating. A store of vitellogenin is already in place, deep in the skin, ready to play its part in the secretion of the female's mating pheromone on her emergence from the den. This vitellogenin was deposited in the skin the preceding year, before hibernation. It was synthesized in the liver and passed into the bloodstream on the way to the ovaries, all in connection with the development of that year's eggs. At that time some of the vitellogenin in the blood was diverted from the circulation to storage in the skin.

Now, vitellogenin is turned into egg yolk by the ovaries, so the more eggs the ovaries produce, the more vitellogenin is demanded from the liver, and the more is passed from the liver into the circulating blood. The total amount of vitellogenin deposited in the skin reflects the overall output of vitellogenin by the liver because as more vitellogenin is formed, more of it is diverted to the skin. The result is a significant relationship. When a female emerges from hibernation this year, the supply of vitellogenin in her skin is directly related to the number of eggs she produced last year. Moreover, the more vitellogenin there is in the skin, the more mating pheromone appears on the female's back. The important final consequence is that females that produced more eggs last year carry more pheromone this year.

This relationship helps explain the observation that males strongly prefer to court large females. Larger snakes are generally older, since snakes continue to grow throughout their lives. Large females also tend to yield more eggs, and, as we have just seen, this translates into more vitellogenin in their skin and more pheromone on their backs the following year. In preferring large females, the male snake is choosing a mate that offers a large amount of mating pheromone and was a prolific egg producer last year. In effect, he opts for proved fecundity and in this way improves his chances of passing on his genes.

The reproductive behavior and pheromones in this garter snake would be intriguing even if this were the end of the story. However, there is one more strange chapter. The red-sided garter snake provides an extraordinary instance of female mimicry that confers a reproductive advantage on certain males. This adaptation first came to the attention of Crews and his students through a census of the mating balls that male snakes form around a female. Out of two hundred mating balls, about 15 percent unexpectedly contained no female snake. Instead, in each case the males were actively courting one particular male snake.

Crews called these males "she-males" and examined a number of them for any traits that might distinguish them from other males. These she-males behaved like normal males in all respects. They courted females as vigorously as did other male snakes, and they did not court ordinary males. Like other males, they preferred to court females rather than she-males in field tests that allowed a free choice between the two. Morphologically there were no discernible differences between males and she-males, but some very interesting biochemical dissimilarities appeared. Like normal males, she-males carried on their backs the female mating pheromone. The proportions were somewhat different from those found in either females or normal males, but the mixture was still active in promoting courtship. Most significantly, these otherwise normal male snakes did not have squalene in their skin lipids. She-males lack the male-recognition pheromone, and it is this that distinguishes them from normal males and leads to their being courted like females. She-males also have a higher concentration of testosterone circulating in their blood, but the significance of this is not yet certain.

However she-males may have acquired their ability to pass themselves off as female snakes, this capability affords them a definite advantage over ordinary males. In competitive field trials Crews released five males and five she-males in an enclosure with an attractive female. In each of 42 tests the snakes formed a mating ball and mating took place. In 29 of these tests (69 precent!) it was a she-male that succeeded in mating with the female snake. The imposters enjoyed a better than two-to-one reproductive advantage over ordinary males.

She-males apparently attain their advantage by distraction. When a she-male joins an established mating ball, some of the males contending for the female interrupt their efforts and start courting the imposter. In the ensuing disturbance and wriggling confusion, the she-male slips into an advantageous position alongside the female. Here he has good chance of becoming the male that wins the female.

Birds

Apart from feathers, birds are structurally much like the reptiles. The similarities, however, do not seem to extend to olfaction and chemical communication. In earlier years even the idea of olfaction in birds was controversial, but it is now well established that birds of some species have a sense of smell.

The evidence for pheromones in birds remains incomplete, although there are some tempting clues. The male mallard duck *Anas platyrhynchos* suffers considerable inhibition of sexual behavior after surgical sectioning of the olfactory nerve, a finding that suggests a role for olfaction in reproduction. Interestingly, the secretion of the the female mallard's uropygial gland changes in chemical composition during the breeding season, although at other times of the year this secretion is similar to that of drakes and ducklings. The uropygial gland is common to nearly all birds and is the source of the oily preen substance that birds apply to their feathers. It is an obvious possible source of a sex attractant or other reproductive signal. We may surmise that the changed preen substance serves as a reproductive pheromone, perhaps attracting the drake or indicating female receptiveness, but so far no experiments have explored these possibilities.

Another line of evidence concerning avian pheromones comes from the group of birds called tubenoses, which includes petrels, albatrosses, and some other species that also live in the open sea. The uropygial glands of these birds produce a large amount of preen substance, enabling the birds to protect their feathers against constant exposure to water. The uropygial secretion of tubenoses has a strong odor to the human nose, and the olfactory system of most of these birds is unusually well developed. Perhaps a search for pheromones in the odoriferous secretions of the tubenoses would be worthwhile, but no investigator has taken up the problem.

One final suggestive clue arises from the fact that the male and female of many species of birds look so much alike that humans can distinguish them only by dissecting the animals. Fortunately the birds themselves have some other means of solving this problem. It is possible that pheromones provide the necessary information, although experiments are lacking here, too.

We have seen that pheromones are probably widespread in fishes and that they have an important place in snakes and salamanders. As in many groups of invertebrates, there have been too few studies to say that chemical communication is absent elsewhere. Many questions and possibilities remain, but it will be some time before a more complete picture is at hand. In contrast, we already know much more concerning chemical communication within mammalian species, and it is to these remaining vertebrates that we now turn.

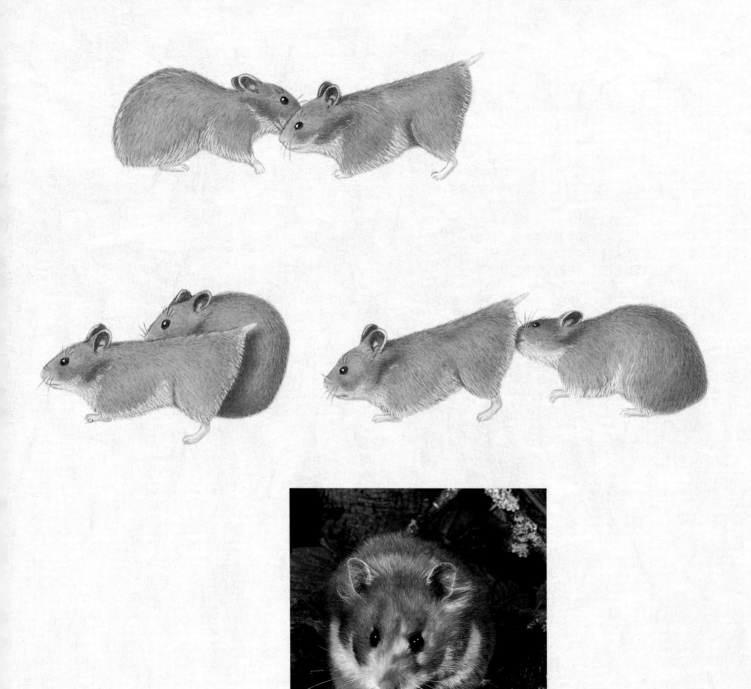

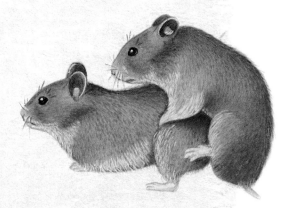

6

MAMMALIAN COMPLEXITIES

■ The golden hamster is so dependent on olfaction for normal mating behavior that a male unable to detect chemical signals will not mate. Pheromones released by a female guide the male through a set mating ritual. First the male approaches the female head-to-head and investigates the skin glands on her head; the female assumes a receptive posture. The male then moves to the female's side and sniffs and licks her flank gland, presumably gaining further information about her reproductive state. He moves again, to the rear of the female, continuing his investigative sniffing and licking. Should he detect a mounting pheromone, he will mount the female and intromit.

The mammals deserve separate consideration in a chapter of their own, as they offer particular problems in the study of chemical communication. From our familiarity with domestic animals we recognize most mammals relatively easily. In addition to the backbone and cranium common to all vertebrates, mammals have hair, they maintain a constant body temperature, the females care for the young and produce milk to nourish them, and, of special interest to us in probing their pheromones, mammals have a well-developed brain. This advanced brain has reached its present extreme in the primates, a collection of almost two hundred species that includes lemurs, monkeys, apes, and man.

With their constant body temperature and enlarged brain, mammals have become relatively independent of their external environment. They can thrive on both land and sea, and unlike reptiles, they can adapt to arctic cold. Although they number only about 4,000 species, mammals have spread over the earth and adopted a remarkable variety of forms. They range in size from the blue whale *Balaenoptera musculus* (the largest animal ever, with the heaviest captured specimen weighing 123,000 kilograms, which equals the weight of 30 elephants!) to the Etruscan shrew *Suncus etruscus* (with a typical weight of 2 grams). There are more than 80 species of dolphins, whales, manatees, and their relatives that are at home in the oceans, and some 950 species of bats that fly in the air. Even the familiar terrestrial animals include forms as varied as anteaters and zebras, porcupines and tigers, baboons and muskrats.

Most mammals are nocturnal and have a highly developed sense of smell. It should be no surprise then that chemical signals, both intra- and interspecific, provide an important part of their information about the world.

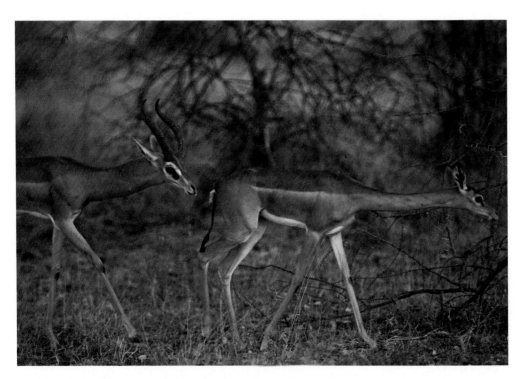

A male East African giraffe-gazelle *Litocranius walleri* sniffs to determine whether the female is sexually receptive.

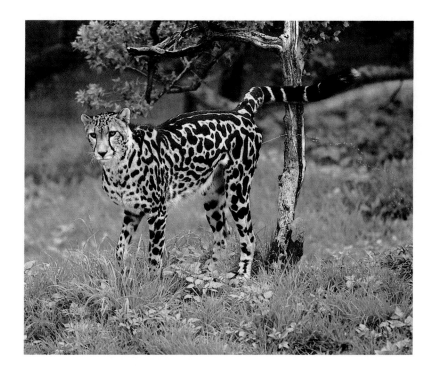

This male king cheetah is marking his territory with a clearly visible jet of urine. The king cheetah is a variant distinguished by black stripes on its back and tail.

Mammals may perceive these signals through the olfactory system or in the vomeronasal organ, which is present and functional in a wide variety of species. Mammals make use of pheromones with functions analogous to those we have seen elsewhere, but they also send many other sorts of chemical messages. These may disclose whether a female is receptive to mating, whether she is lactating, or whether she is pregnant. They may lead to the recognition of individuals or discriminate subordinate from dominant animals. They may distinguish between the sexes or among members of specific colonies or age groups. An individual, family, or pack may mark its territory, leaving a line of chemical flags that indicate boundaries just as clearly for its species as surveyors'

monuments do for us. Other signals lead to physiological changes in the recipient. There are pheromones that accelerate or decelerate puberty in immature females, pheromones that influence the timing of the estrous cycle, and pheromones that cause a male to mount a receptive female.

The chemical signals of mammals are carried in a wide variety of secretions and excretions; particularly important are urine, feces, and the products of glands in the skin. Other members of the species may pick up these scents by sniffing or licking an individual, or an animal may deposit a signal on the ground or on other surfaces in the environment. Often specific behaviors disseminate these signals. Hippopotamuses *(Hippopotamus amphibius)*

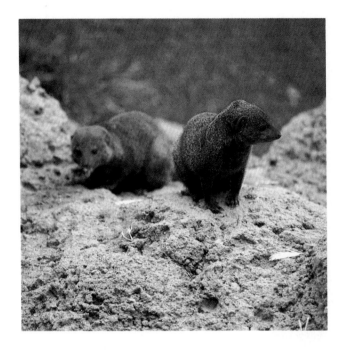

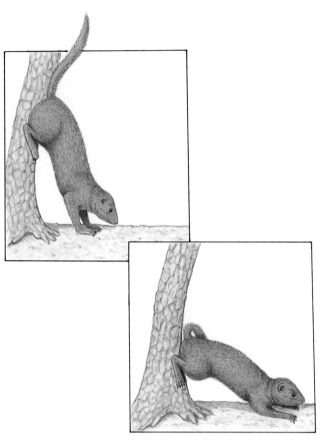

The dwarf mongoose is a small carnivore native to the open savannah of eastern and southern Africa. It leaves its mark by performing a handstand in front of a vertical object, then rubbing its anal gland down the object.

wag their tails as they urinate, sending a spray of urine over nearby plants. The male cheetah *Acinonyx jubatus* and other male cats squirt urine backward onto sprigs of vegetation and other conspicuous objects. Dwarf mongooses *(Helogale parvula)* do a handstand in front of an upright object that they then mark by dragging their anal gland downward over the objcct. Saddle-back tamarins *(Saguinus fuscicollis)* straddle or sprawl on an object to mark it with their suprapubic gland.

Complexities to Unravel

Our understanding of the biology and chemistry of these mammalian pheromones is limited, in large measure because of the complexity of mammalian life and the mammalian brain. In many mammals the enlarged brain incorporates highly evolved structures associated with perception of sight, sound, and touch, as well as taste and odor, and the ability of mammals to integrate information received by these various senses enormously complicates efforts to understand any specific signal. Dietland Müller-Schwarze, of the College of Environmental Science and Forestry of the State University of New York, has long studied behavior and pheromones in deer. Twenty years ago Müller-Schwarze noted that when a black-tailed deer *(Odocoileus hemionus columbianus)* is alarmed, it alerts other nearby deer by releasing a garliclike odor from the metatarsal glands on the outer surface of its hind legs. At the same time it gives visual cues by erection of its tail and anal hair, by cocking its ears, and by walking with a stiff-legged gait. It also provides auditory signals by hissing and stamping its forefeet on the ground. How are we to sort out whether other deer respond to any *one* of these simultaneous visual, auditory, and chemical cues? In this regard it is worth noting that deer are not laboratory animals, and that even seemingly simple experiments to explore a question of this sort can be tricky to carry out.

Even if a signal involves only a single sense, interpreting the reaction it elicits can present difficulties for the investigator studying mammals. A large brain leads to behavior that is complex and not necessarily reproducible. Sometimes, a mammal that receives a pheromonal signal may have no observable response. Perhaps it is ignoring the signal, or perhaps it has learned something from the signal and stored it away for future use. Responses may reflect what has been learned in the past; elements from prior experience may influence how a mammal reacts.

Other species, including sea slugs and other invertebrates, also exhibit learning. But, if you pinch three sea slugs *(Navanax inermis)* on the back, it is likely that each one will recoil and secrete its yellow alarm pheromone. This behavior is built into *N. inermis* at a fundamental level. If you pinch three dogs on the back, it is much less certain what may happen. One dog may bite you, one may growl, and one may run away. Furthermore, there is no assurance that the next time you pinch the same dogs each one will react as it did before. Responses to pheromonal signals can be similarly unpredictable and irreproducible, and it may be difficult to identify either signal or response. The very notion of a specific reaction to a given signal may become a misleading simplification. This is a different world from that of invertebrates or simpler vertebrates.

The Coolidge Effect

A related problem with mammals is habituation; that is, the response of a mammal to a given stimulus often decreases on repetition. As the stimulus loses novelty, the receiver may simply disregard it. An example of this behavior is the Coolidge effect, which the following experiment illustrates. An investigator places a male and a receptive female in an enclosure, and allows the male to mate with the female until the male expresses no further interest in mating. The investigator then removes the mated, but still receptive, female and replaces her with a new receptive female. The jaded male reacts with rekindled interest, and he mates with the new female. This effect is typical of a variety of mammals. The possibility of habituation has to be kept in mind in interpreting mammalian behavior and in designing bioassays for pheromones and other stimuli.

There has been discussion, both pro and con, in the behavioral literature concerning extrapolation of the Coolidge effect to the analysis of human philandering. This delicate issue lies outside our present domain, but it is perhaps appropriate to point out the curious origin of the term "Coolidge effect." Most such designations honor the discoverer of a phenomenon or a significant contributor to its investigation. The Coolidge effect, however, takes its name from Calvin Coolidge, the thirtieth president of the United States (1923–1929) and a man who had an invincible reputation for small-town New England rectitude. More precisely, the Coolidge effect takes its name from the following story about the president and his wife.

It seems that President and Mrs. Coolidge were visiting a government farm, where they were warmly greeted and then taken on separate tours of the premises. When Mrs. Coolidge was shown the large chicken coop, the resident rooster was pointed out and she was told that he copulated frequently throughout the day. "Oh, really?" she said. "You must be sure to tell that to the President." The President arrived later at the chicken coop on his own tour, and he was duly informed of the rooster's activities. "Always with the same hen?" the President asked slowly. "Oh no, Mr. President," came the reply, "with a different hen each time." The President nodded thoughtfully and responded, "You must be sure to tell that to Mrs. Coolidge."

Behaviorists are quick to point out that the name is a misnomer, as the story does not quite fit the effect. The fabled rooster had free access to many females at all times, while the Coolidge effect concerns a male presented sequentially with two receptive females. The name has stuck, however, and is now standard in the literature of animal behavior.

Interactions and Other Obstacles

There is another complexity that is not unique to mammals but is a particular problem for investigators studying mammalian chemical communication. One signal may modify, enhance, or influence the recipient's response to another signal. In discussing both ants and honey bees, we spoke briefly of the interaction of chemical signals with other sensory information. This interaction is widespread in mammals. A pretty example that involves a physiological reaction comes from observations on the golden hamster *Mesocricetus auratus* made by John G. Vandenbergh of the Department of Zoology at North Carolina State University, an investigator who has made many significant contributions to our understanding of mammalian reproductive pheromones.

Hamsters breed seasonally, and the male's gonads shrink and regrow with the changing seasons. When male hamsters are exposed to short days and long nights, their testes become smaller, and this effect is reversed by long days and short nights. Vandenbergh noted that the testes regrow more rapidly with long days if the males are exposed at the same time to cages that have been soiled by receptive female hamsters. Some signal, presumably a pheromone left behind by the females, acts to enhance the reaction to long days. The male gonads regrow appreciably faster when the males receive both the chemical signal from the females and the visual signal of a lengthened day. It is easy to see how an unsuspected interaction of this sort can complicate the interpretation of behavior and the design of valid bioassays.

Another obstacle to the analysis of chemical communication in mammals is the *chemical* complexity of many mammalian pheromones, and we will have more to say about this later. For the time being, note that chemical signals in mammals differ from those we have examined before. These messages are not necessarily urgent. The responses they elicit may result from the integration of the signal with other information and may be variable. Learning may play a critical role in associating scent, situation, and response. Certain investigators have thought that these differences render the unmodified term *pheromone* inappropriate for describing mammalian chemical signals. Some have preferred a new designation, such as *social odors*, for these mammalian signals; many others, while retaining the established term *pheromone* for its convenience, have been careful to point out the many distinctions between chemical signals in invertebrates and mammals.

All this has meant that progress in piecing together a detailed understanding of many mammalian pheromones has been slow. It has been difficult to move from observed behavior to the chemistry of the implicated signals and their biological significance. The dog *Canis familiaris* and its pheromones are good examples. Dogs and humans have been living together for at least eight or ten thousand years, and early on humans must have discovered that a bitch in heat attracts male dogs by her smell. Although this may have been one of the first pheromones in another species noticed by man, there is no agreement yet on the chemistry of the signal. For a few years a compound isolated from the vagina of receptive bitches was thought to be responsible for the attraction of males. Another, more carefully designed investigation revealed, however, that this was not the case. In the second study, dogs reacted to suitable controls just as reliably as to test samples of the putative pheromone.

Similarly, there is probably no marking behavior better known to humans than a dog, with hind leg raised against lamppost or tree, delivering a burst of urine to celebrate his passing. The signal he leaves interests other dogs mightily, but we have little idea about what chemicals are implicated or what it all means. (This is an instance in which ignorance cannot be traced to a shortage of material to examine. The ecological literature offers the estimate that in New York City alone, dogs annually deposit up to four million liters of urine and 18,000 metric tons of feces. It is safe to assume that essentially all of this material goes to waste.)

Another example comes from the domestic cow *Bos taurus*. Chemical signals affect the reproductive behavior of cows, and humans would probably find considerable economic advantage in understanding some of these signals in detail. Artificial insemination is a mainstay in raising cattle for market, but the cow can become pregnant only if inseminated when she is receptive. Cattlemen would like a dependable indication of the cow's breeding condition. Unfortunately, despite substantial efforts, the chemical signals that disclose a cow's reproductive status to a bull remain unintelligible to humans.

All of this is not to say that we have no good behavioral and chemical information about mammalian signals. There is, however, much more behavioral work than chemical. There are a few systems in which we have a reasonable understanding of both the chemical composition of a signal and the response it produces, but there are many others in which the pieces of the puzzle do not yet fit together. We shall look at a sample of pheromones in mammals to get an idea of our present knowledge here. In the same way that mammalian pheromones pose special difficulties in comparison with those of other vertebrates, human pheromones offer unique problems in comparison with those of other mammals, and we shall postpone consideration of humans until the following chapter.

Pheromones of the Black-Tailed Deer

The artiodactyls are the hoofed mammals with an even number of toes, such as sheep, camels, and giraffes, and the deer are one part of this group. The black-tailed deer *Odocoileus hemionus columbianus* is a relatively small mule deer native to British Columbia, Washington, and Oregon. Like other related deer, it possesses a gland in the skin covering part of its ankle on the inside of its hind leg. This is known as the tarsal gland, and it is made conspicuous by a tuft of bright, stiff hairs. We previously mentioned the metatarsal gland found on the outside of the hind leg of this animal and the observation that it produces an alarm pheromone. The functions of both

these glands remained obscure until Müller-Schwarze's investigations. These problems first attracted his interest when, as a graduate student, he observed deer in the Black Forest of southern Germany and wondered why they had scent-producing skin glands. His pioneering studies of the black-tailed deer were the first investigations to combine behavioral studies with the chemical analysis of a vertebrate pheromone.

We now appreciate that the scent of the tarsal gland is crucial in a number of ways to the social behavior of black-tailed deer. Members of an established herd check each other's tarsal glands regularly, sniffing and licking at the tuft of hairs, so that during the day each individual is examined once or twice an hour. At night, checking is even more frequent. A strange deer that comes into a herd is exam-

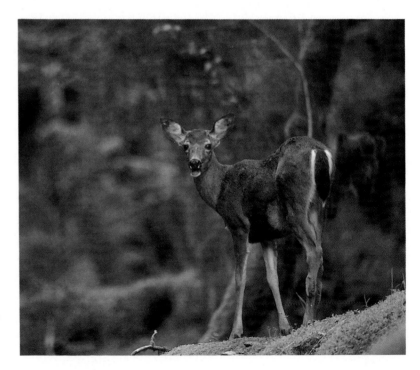

A black-tailed deer in the rain forest of the Olympic National Park in Washington.

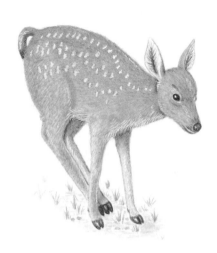

$CH_3CH_2CH_2CH_2CH_2CH_2CH_2CH_2HC$

Dihydro deer lactone

Deer lactone

E-Deer lactone

A male black-tailed deer fawn brings its hind legs together to rub-urinate.

Bioassays establish that the *Z* double bond is important for the attractivity of the deer lactone. The compound with the *E* double bond is only weakly attractive. The compound with a single bond instead of a double bond does not attract black-tailed deer.

ined repeatedly, although the stranger does not approach and sniff the herd members. Smelling the tarsal gland is the first stage in aggressive behavior and also the means by which a fawn recognizes its mother.

Besides sniffing and licking, the other significant behavior involving the tarsal gland is "rub-urination." A deer brings its hind legs together, releases a jet of urine onto the tarsal tufts, and then rubs the left and right tarsal glands against each other. Fawns begin doing this as early as the second day of life, and it is common in deer of either sex and all ages in a variety of situations. Two bucks will rub-urinate when threatening each other, and fawns will do so when distressed. Several other species of deer display similar behavior.

Müller-Schwarze and R. M. Silverstein (whose work with bark beetles we noted earlier) and their co-workers found that the tarsal tufts carry a complex mixture of volatile compounds. From this mixture they isolated the major component, and they determined the structure of this "deer lactone." They then synthesized this compound in the laboratory and demonstrated that it is the constituent of the tarsal extract most effective in eliciting sniffing and licking. In one of their bioassays, they sprayed solutions of various concentrations of the deer lactone, or of crude extract of tarsal tufts, or of control substances onto the outside of the hind leg of a deer. Other deer approached this animal and sniffed and licked at the applied material. The time spent in these activities supplied a measure of the material's attractivity.

Müller-Schwarze and Silverstein next investigated the origin of the deer lactone. Was it a direct secretion of the tarsal gland or a component of urine that reached that area only through rub-urination? The scientists explored this question by first cleaning the surface of the tarsal gland and then squeezing out and collecting its contents. They found no deer lactone in the secretion obtained this way. However, in clean urine they did find the lactone in a concentration greater than 1 milligram per liter. This then is the source of the attractant.

It is worth noting this concentration of about 1 milligram per liter. On the generous assumption that a deer squirts 10 milliliters of urine on its tarsal glands as it rubs its legs together, we can calculate that only about 10 micrograms of the deer lactone is transferred to serve as an attractant. This compound is, however, the principal constituent of the volatiles obtained on extraction of the tarsal tufts. It is not unusual for mammalian urine, feces, and glandular secretions to contain literally hundreds of volatile substances and for many of them to be present in very low concentration. Although the attractant is the principal volatile compound isolated in this case, there is in general no reliable correlation between concentration and pheromonal activity. The substance responsible for a particular signal of interest may be a minor constituent of a complex mixture.

We spoke of "clean urine" in the last paragraph. Many animals excrete urine contaminated by secretions that are added after the urine leaves the bladder but before it is finally discharged. An investigator can obtain uncontaminated urine from laboratory animals merely by inserting a catheter and drawing urine directly from the bladder. Getting clean urine from black-tailed deer, however, is less convenient. These investigators got their first sample of urine for isolation of the deer lactone by patiently watching and stalking a deer until it urinated on a patch of fresh snow. Then they scooped up the snow and dispatched it to the laboratory for analysis. Later they collected samples of clean urine by catheter from anesthetized deer.

Once we know that the deer lactone comes from the bladder, we can see a function for rub-urination. This stereotyped behavior is an indispensable step in moving the deer lactone from the urine onto the surface of the tarsal glands, where it acts as an attractant for other deer. As rub-urination and examination of the tarsal glands are a part of so many activities for these deer, we may guess that other compounds, perhaps many others, carried on the tarsal tufts must also convey information. Judging from the variety of situations in which the tarsal tufts are checked, we can surmise that these messages pertain to matters of social organization, such as individual identity, herd membership, and position of dominance or subordination in the group. The compounds bearing these messages could originate in the secretion of the tarsal gland, in the urine, or in secretions added to the urine. It appears that a deer approaches, sniffs, and licks the tarsal tufts of another animal primarily in response to the odor of the deer lactone, and that these other compounds, perhaps first encountered during this sniffing and licking, transmit the messages of interest. Detailed information about these diverse social signals is still lacking.

Flehmen

Other types of behavior in black-tailed deer also appear to be associated with pheromones. There are skin glands in the tail, and deer will sniff one another's and their own tails when excited. There are glands in the forehead that they rub against twigs and branches in a marking behavior. Other deer will sniff and lick such marks with evident interest. The hooves also carry scent glands, and the footprints left by an animal running to escape danger attract attention from other deer. Another pheromonal reaction, which is shared with many other species, is the lip-curl response or flehmen. Cats, ungulates, bats, marsupials, and some other mammals show this striking behavior.

Müller-Schwarze and Silverstein studied flehmen in these deer. Flehmen is primarily a reaction of male mammals to female urine, and in most species only direct physical contact with the urine will trigger it. First the animal sniffs the urine, then licks it, and takes it into his mouth. He curls his upper lip, parts

his jaws, and raises his head, turning it from side to side or nodding up and down, depending on the species. The animal breathes deeply. This intriguing behavior moves the urine from the mouth and tongue into the vomeronasal organ. Flehmen was formally described in 1930 and had been familiar to farmers and others who handled animals long before that, but it remains poorly understood. (Flehmen is the only standard behavioral term for this action. The word is originally German, but its origin is uncertain.)

Only male black-tailed deer commonly exhibit flehmen, and they do so only during the breeding season from late September to early January. At this time the males respond to urine from males, females, or fawns equally readily. Flehmen is largely species-specific, although black-tailed deer do react weakly to the urine of the white-tailed deer *Odocoileus*

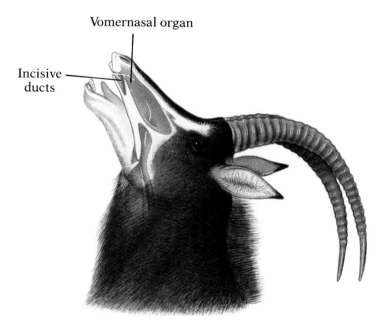

Vomernasal organ

Incisive ducts

A male sable antelope *Hippotragus niger* gives a flehmen response to female urine. The vomeronasal organ of some species, including deer and antelopes, connects with passages known as the incisive ducts, which open just below the nostrils and also communicate directly with the nose and mouth. This arrangement may permit both airborne odorants and molecules carried in liquid from the mouth to enter the vomeronasal organ.

A male mule deer *Odocoileus hemionus* performs flehmen. The mule deer is a very close relative of the black-tailed deer but is native to the broad area from southern Alaska to northern Mexico.

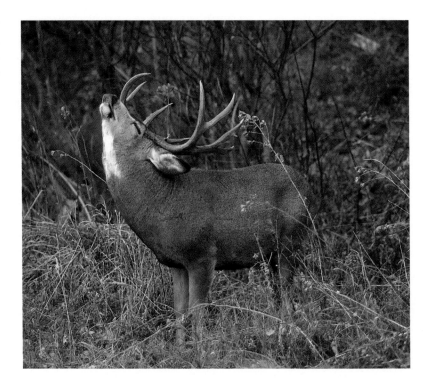

virginianus and the goat *Capra hircus.* After exhibiting flehmen, both the performing male and other nearby deer typically return to routine activities, such as feeding. Presumably the signal in the urine is evaluated after it is detected in the vomeronasal organ, but the deer exhibit no characteristic behavior and flehmen has no overt consequence.

Neither the deer lactone nor other urinary constituents that have been identified induce flehmen, but we do now know some of the chemical properties of the effective signal. Müller-Schwarze and Silverstein have fractionated deer urine and followed the activity using a flehmen bioassay. From this work it appears that the deer are reacting to a compound or mixture of compounds that is water-soluble, heat-stable, and relatively nonvolatile. It could

be as large as a small protein. The chemical characterization of this material requires further attention, as does the significance of flehmen for the deer. At present we know that the urine of black-tailed deer contains at least two different signals, the deer lactone, which is detected in the olfactory system, and the signal prompting flehmen, which is detected in the vomeronasal organ and the accessory olfactory system. Many other mammals also use both systems to detect chemical signals.

The black-tailed deer has provided us with our first indication that a chemical signal can be associated with an individual rather than an entire species. The fawn recognizes its mother by investigating her tarsal gland. The implication is that each doe has a different signal and that the fawn can pick out one of these. Such signals are often called recognition pheromones, and their existence suggests a level of complexity that we have not met before. We shall have more to say about recognition pheromones a little later.

A Sex Pheromone in the Pig's Saliva

The swine make up another subgroup of artiodactyls, and these animals include creatures such as the bush pig and the warthog, as well as the domestic pig *Sus scrofa*. Not only has the pig been of agricultural importance for thousands of years, but it has attained a substantial modern position as a laboratory animal, notably in a miniature version that was derived through selective breeding about forty years ago. Pigs have served as useful subjects for experimental cardiovascular surgery and for the study of atherosclerosis and radiation damage, among other things. However, it is really the pig's status as a farm animal that has led to our knowledge of its salivary sex pheromone. This is a rare mammalian example of a simple signal with a fairly reliable response.

In the presence of a mature boar, most receptive sows assume an immobile posture with the back down and ears cocked. In this position, which is called lordosis, the sow will allow the boar to mount and mate. We know that seeing, hearing, and smelling the boar all contribute to lordosis, and that the odor of the boar is especially significant. Boars have a musky breath, and the compounds that are responsible for this and for the pheromonal action of boar scent can be isolated from their saliva. These compounds are two steroids closely related to the male sex hormone testosterone. One of these compounds has a thor-

oughly disagreeable and urinelike odor, while the odor of the other is more pleasant. These two steroids are also present in boar fat and are responsible for the offensive taste and odor known as boar taint that sometimes ruin cooked boar meat. Both compounds are synthesized in the testes and stored largely in the salivary glands. Chemical signals in saliva are unusual, but there are scattered reports of them in several other mammals as well.

This pheromone has attained practical importance among pig farmers because, as with cattle, artificial insemination is a major commercial technique of pig breeding. Here again the breeder must know when a female is receptive in order to inseminate her at the optimum time for fertilization. A technician can evaluate a sow presented for artificial insemination by pressing down on her back and watching her reaction. If the sow responds with lordosis, she is judged to be receptive and ready for insemination. About two-thirds of the sows that respond to the pressure test and are then inseminated become pregnant and bear a litter of pigs. A failing of the procedure is that 30 percent or more of sows that actually are in estrus (the fertile period of their reproductive cycle) fail to respond to pressure, so that many fertilizable animals are not identified for insemination.

Some years ago a team of British government veterinarians made a discovery with important repercussions for the routine artificial insemination of pigs. They demonstrated that about half of the estrous sows that are initially unresponsive to the back-pressure test do respond to pressure after being sprayed on the snout with a solution of boar salivary pheromone. After artificial insemination these treated sows produce litters at the same rate as sows that respond to the pressure without the pheromone. This simple technique, now exploited commercially, increases pig production appreciably. An aerosol preparation containing the steroid pheromone has been successfully marketed under the trade name "Boar Mate," the first mammalian pheromone to achieve recognition in the marketplace.

Attracting the Male Hamster

More than one-third of the described mammals are rodents, and these are the most common mammals not only in numbers of species but in numbers of individuals as well. Most of these rodents belong to a huge group that includes rats, mice, gerbils, and similar species. One of these is the Syrian golden hamster *Mesocricetus auratus*, a native of the desert that has considerable standing as an experimental animal. Oddly, all the golden hamsters now held in laboratories around the world are descended from one family, a mother and twelve young, that were gathered near Aleppo and brought out of Syria in 1930.

This species of hamster has been especially prominent in studies of reproductive pheromones owing to its unusual dependence on olfaction for normal sexual behavior. A male golden hamster that cannot detect chemical signals fails to respond to receptive females. Because the normal male is so dependent on his nose and vomeronasal organ, scientists have been able to avoid some complexity normally associated with investigations of mammalian pheromones.

Some years ago, my research group at The Rockefeller University became interested in investigating the chemistry of hamster reproductive signals. My colleagues Carl Pfaffmann and Robert J. O'Connell were studying the hamster's reproductive behavior, and they encouraged us to join them in a chemical study. It was already well established that the female hamster ordinarily engages in a marking be-

havior every four days, just before coming into estrus. In their native setting these hamsters lead solitary lives, and when she has no young, the female lives alone in an underground burrow. We can imagine that in the desert she goes forth on the night before estrus and lays a trail to attract a male. He responds to the attractant, following the trail to the female's burrow. She awaits him within. In the laboratory the female hamster leaves a trail by dragging her hindquarters along the floor of her cage and depositing a watery liquid secreted from the vagina. This vaginal discharge contains a number of pheromonal signals for the male, including one that is a

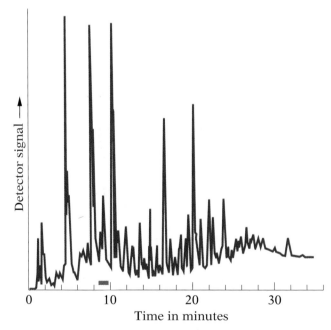

A gas chromatogram of volatile compounds isolated from the vaginal discharge of the golden hamster. The bar under the chromatogram indicates a fraction that was attractive to male hamsters in the bioassay; from this fraction dimethyl disulfide was later isolated.

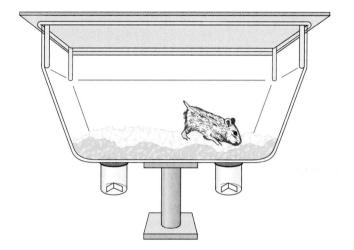

The bioassay for the hamster attractant makes use of a cage with two clusters of holes drilled in the bottom and covered with wire mesh. Under each set of holes is attached the perforated metal top of a small screw-cap jar. In carrying out the bioassay the investigator places a control sample on a piece of filter paper in one jar and the fraction to be tested on a piece of filter paper in the other, and then screws the jars onto the caps fixed below the cage. The samples now diffuse up through the perforated caps, into the cage, and to the hamster.

potent attractant, but the chemistry of these signals was completely unexplored.

The chemistry of this attractant pheromone was the first problem that Alan G. Singer undertook when he joined us at Rockefeller as a postdoctoral fellow. His gas chromatographic examination of the volatile material from the vaginal discharge gave a chromatogram with more than 85 peaks. Each peak in the chromatogram represents at least one substance, and in many cases three or four, so there are probably more than two hundred volatile compounds in this mixture.

As we have seen before, successful isolation of pheromones demands careful fractionation and a sensitive bioassay. Our collaborator Robert O'Connell designed and conducted a very dependable bioassay for Singer's fractionation of these volatiles. For the bioassay O'Connell modified a hamster cage so that odors from both a test sample and a control substance diffused into the cage from jars placed underneath, on opposite sides of the cage. The male hamster was frequently resting when a bioassay began. If the sample was the unmodified vaginal discharge, the hamster would rouse himself and, following the attractant gradient, move to the spot in the cage over the test jar. There he would begin sniffing and digging up the bedding, apparently trying to reach the source of the pheromone. He responded in other tests with similar or diminished enthusiasm, depending on the sample under study. The time he spent sniffing and digging, as well as the time that elapsed before he began to respond, furnished measures of the attractivity of the sample.

Using O'Connell's bioassay, Singer learned that none of the major volatile components, represented by the largest peaks in the chromatogram, was attractive. Very active material, however, was located in the region marked with the short bar on the chromatogram. Repurification, retesting, and finally mass spectrometric analysis revealed that the attractive substance was dimethyl disulfide

(CH_3SSCH_3). This is a simple, well-known compound that has an appalling stench in bulk. We all encounter it in trace amounts as a constituent of the complex aromas of many foodstuffs: broccoli, beer, and liver, among others. Under these circumstances it is not conspicuous or offensive.

Hamsters, like humans, prefer dimethyl disulfide in limited doses. Using calibrated gas chromatography, Singer found that the vaginal discharge collected from each female hamster contained about 5 nanograms of dimethyl disulfide. This is a minute amount, but it turns out to be vastly more than is needed to draw the attention of a male hamster. As little as 0.05 picogram of dimethyl disulfide placed in the test jar produced about twice as great a response in the bioassay as did a control sample. As larger samples of dimethyl disulfide are tested, the hamster's sniffing and digging first increase and then level off. When samples consist of more than about 50 picograms, dimethyl disulfide ceases to become more attractive. Even these small amounts are large relative to the hamster's threshold sensitivity to the pheromone. Note that the amounts are material placed in the jar, not the amounts that reach the hamster's nose. In the bioassay only a very small portion of the material diffuses out of the jar and up into the cage. Most of it remains in the jar throughout the test, dissolved in the solvent employed to prepare the sample. The hamster must be reacting to an amount of attractant several orders of magnitude less than the quantity in the jar. Taking all the pertinent factors into consideration and making some reasonable and conservative assumptions, we calculated that the initial perception by the hamster probably required fewer than two hundred molecules of dimethyl disulfide. This sensitivity to a pheromone was unprecedented in a mammal.

In the bioassay, appropriate concentrations of dimethyl disulfide evoked about 60 percent as much sniffing and digging as did the vaginal discharge, indicating that the complete pheromonal signal may contain more components. Singer isolated a number of inactive compounds from the natural secretion, but no other attractive constituents could be identified. Even when dimethyl disulfide is combined with large fractions of the discharge, the mixture is always less attractive than the total discharge. This probably means that the combined odor of most or all of the other volatiles in the vaginal discharge is responsible for the greater attractivity of the total discharge. If this is correct, the search for other attractive compounds fails because a grand mixture of components is required for the missing activity. Such complex odors resulting from many substances are often significant in mammalian pheromones, and we shall return to them when we discuss pheromones in the mouse.

More Signals from the Same Source

For the moment we want to continue following Singer's exploration of hamster pheromones. After identifying dimethyl disulfide as an attractant, he turned his attention to another property of the vaginal discharge. There are signals here that mediate a number of other behavioral and physiological actions, such as male exploration of the female genital area, reduction of male aggression toward the female, and rapid elevation of the level of testosterone in the male's blood.

There were also intriguing reports from other studies of golden hamsters concerning a pheromone that elicits male copulatory behavior. As with the attractant, there were good behavioral descriptions of this signal, but absolutely nothing was known about its chemistry. This pheromone acts on the male only at the end of his ritual of exploring a receptive female. In this exploration, he typically approaches the female and begins to sniff and lick her about the ears and head, where there are skin glands that presumably yield information concerning her reproductive status. A receptive female soon assumes an immobile lordosis posture akin to that of the estrous sow. The male moves to her side and investigates her flank gland, which is a skin gland of ill-defined function found in both sexes. He sniffs and licks here, too. Finally, he moves to the rear and investigates the vaginal region in the same fashion. First he sniffs and licks, and then very soon, he mounts and intromits. This final sequence of events suggests the presence of a pheromone that elicits copulation.

Experiments with female surrogates provided encouraging support for this idea. If an inert, anesthetized male is propped up on his four legs in an imitation of the lordosis posture in the cage of a normal test male, the test male will give this strange immobile object a cursory examination and then ignore it. However, if the hindquarters of the anesthetized male have been painted with vaginal discharge, the response is quite different. This object now captures the test male's full attention. He investigates, moves to the rear of the anesthetized animal, sniffs and licks the discharge, mounts, and attempts to intromit. He mounts this surrogate female only after sniffing and licking the painted hindquarters, and this behavior lends further support to the idea that a signal in the discharge stimulates mounting and copulation.

We called this signal the mounting pheromone, and Singer's efforts next turned to its isolation and identification. As no one knew anything about the chemistry of aphrodisiac pheromones, we were enthusiastic at the prospect of unique discoveries. We undertook this new problem with the indispensable collabora-

tion and encouragement of Foteos Macrides, a neurobiologist at the Worcester Foundation for Experimental Biology, and his research group. Macrides created a bioassay for the mounting pheromone from the surrogate-female experiment just described. An investigator applied fractions of the vaginal discharge to the hindquarters of an anesthetized male and determined their activity. For a semiquantitative measure of the test sample's aphrodisiac activity, the investigator counted the number of distinct attempts at intromission made by a test male during a five-minute exposure to the stimulus sample. The Worcester group also maintained the hamster colony and regularly collected vaginal discharge from females for Singer's isolation work. This was in addition to their own research into the detection of the mounting pheromone that we will come to shortly.

The first venture in isolating the mounting pheromone was a complete failure. Naturally enough, Singer initially tested the activity of the entire mixture of volatiles from which dimethyl disulfide had been obtained. To our surprise, the volatiles were totally inactive. When they were distilled out from the vaginal discharge, all the activity remained in the nonvolatile residue. Furthermore, preliminary separations quickly showed that, regardless of the method of fractionation, the large molecules always appeared to elicit the mounting activity. The mounting pheromone appeared to be large and nonvolatile, and at the time these were puzzling properties for a mammalian pheromone.

Everyone knew that insect pheromones were relatively small molecules and volatile. It had seemed reasonable that mammalian pheromones should be the same. Indeed, the deer lactone, the boar salivary signal, and the hamster attractant were all familiar by this time, and all were volatile. Our own knowledge of the vomeronasal organ was still rudimentary, and it would be some time before the idea of a nonvolatile pheromone made sense. Discovery of these unexpected gross properties of the mounting pheromone, however, had an immediate practical effect. Gas chromatographic techniques had been the key to isolation of dimethyl disulfide, and we had foreseen continuing this approach in searching for the mounting pheromone. However, gas chromatography is applicable only to volatile substances and would be totally useless for handling nonvolatile materials. To find the mounting pheromone, Singer first had to train himself in methods for purifying large molecules. This he did without delay.

Once he had mastered these procedures, Singer found that aphrodisiac activity was associated with a fraction of small proteins from the vaginal discharge. The next major step was the most significant one in the entire investigation. Singer was able to isolate and purify a single active protein. This substance was the major protein constituent of the discharge, and 10 micrograms of it, about one-tenth the amount contained in a single collection of discharge from one female, had aphrodisiac activity comparable to that of the whole discharge. This new protein accounted for all the mounting activity, and other similar proteins in the discharge were devoid of activity. Singer's persistent efforts had led to the isolation and characterization of a quite unexpected substance, a proteinaceous mammalian pheromone. It received the name aphrodisin.

We can deal now with the puzzle of a nonvolatile pheromone. By the time the detailed chemical characterization of aphrodisin was unfolding at Rockefeller, we appreciated how a nonvolatile substance might function as a pheromone. Documentation was gathering that the vomeronasal organ is the site of detection of several vertebrate pheromones that regulate hormone levels, aggression, and aspects of sexual behavior. It was also now indisputable that nonvolatile substances could be transported to the vomeronasal organ in liquids from the mouth or snout. These discoveries made it attractive to postulate that aphrodisin was detected not by the olfactory system, but by the vomeronasal organ and accessory olfactory system. Macrides then made the critical experimental connection between the vomeronasal organ and aphrodisin: he showed that the male hamster responded to the mounting pheromone only if he had a functional vomeronasal organ. The earlier mystery of a nonvolatile pheromone vanished, and for organisms possessing a vomeronasal organ the supposition that pheromones were necessarily volatile faded away.

A nonvolatile aphrodisiac offers unmistakable biological advantages. Unlike a pheromone that attracts the male from a distance, the message carried by aphrodisin is germane only in the immediate vicinity of a receptive female. An aphrodisiac disseminated on the breeze throughout a population of male hamsters could spread chaos and havoc. In fact, however, the male must be in direct physical contact with the vaginal discharge for the pheromone to be transferred to his snout, moved into the vomeronasal organ, and detected. The pheromone triggers his mounting reaction only in a suitable context.

Optimizing the Timing of Sexual Maturity

One of the best-known rodents is *Mus musculus*, the ubiquitous house mouse. As represented by inbred strains and commonly known as the laboratory mouse, this species has been more studied by scientists than any other vertebrate species. *M. musculus* also occupies a special place in the history of mammalian

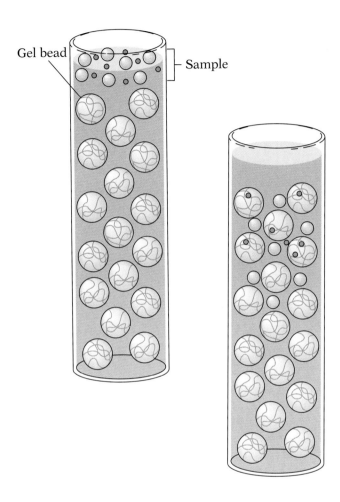

Gel bead

Sample

Gel filtration chromatography is one important method for separating protein molecules of different size. The gel beads contain pores too small for the larger (red) molecules to enter, but large enough to accommodate the smaller (blue) ones. When an investigator passes a mixture of red and blue molecules through the column of gel beads, the blue molecules are held up in the pores and thus move more slowly. As a result, the red molecules pass through the column more rapidly and emerge before the blue ones. In this way the investigator can obtain fractions of pure red molecules and pure blue molecules.

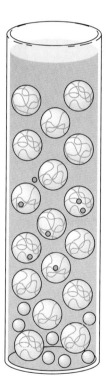

pheromones. After the work on bombykol, the sex attractant of the silkworm moth, had become widely appreciated and chemical communication was attracting enthusiastic attention, the greatest stimulus to searching for pheromones in mammals came from studies on mice.

By 1959 scientists recognized that social cues of some sort had a significant role in the reproductive behavior of the mouse. To some extent, the events of the estrous cycle and pregnancy in any one mouse were under the influence of other mice. The presence of a group of females, for example, slowed down

An adult house mouse with its young. The house mouse has accompanied human beings everywhere and thrives in human habitats all over the earth.

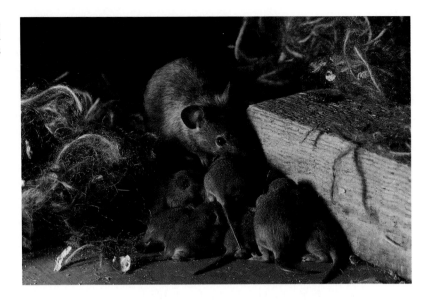

the estrous cycle of a female, while the presence of a male mouse accelerated it. Equally surprising, if a recently inseminated female was exposed to a strange male, her fertilized eggs failed to implant in the uterus. Instead of commencing pregnancy in the usual fashion, she returned to her estrous cycle. Scientists soon learned that odors from the urine of the male and female mice were responsible for these remarkable effects. This meant that mice used reproductive pheromones, and scientists naturally wondered whether the same was true of other mammals.

These signals in mouse urine furnish us a second instance of a pheromone associated with an individual rather than a species. Exposing the female mouse to urine from a strange male terminates her pregnancy. Urine from the male that inseminated her does not have this effect. Somehow, the female distinguishes the odor of her recent partner's urine from that of other males.

A short time after the discovery of mouse pheromones, scientists learned that the timing of puberty in a young female mouse—that is, her initial ovulation—is also affected by other mice. Urine from a group of females can postpone puberty, and urine from a male can advance it. If a young female is exposed to urine from both females and a male at the same time, the pheromone from the females initially overrides the male signal, but as the young female matures, the male signal becomes controlling.

We can speculate that for wild mice such extraordinary outside control over puberty is advantageous. In her family unit a pheromone from a young female's mother and sisters protects her from early puberty and insemination by her father or some other male. If the young female remains with the family, she gradually loses this safeguard as she reaches adulthood. If she leaves home for new surroundings away from mother and sisters, her protection quickly vanishes. In either setting, she eventually reaches puberty and is ready for mating and reproduction. Should an adult male appear on the scene before her natural maturity, he can induce her puberty straightaway and then mate with her. Two of the scientists who assembled the evidence for these effects are F. H. Bronson, of the University of Texas, and John G. Vandenbergh, whom we have mentioned earlier. Both remain active investigators in this area.

Mouse urine also contains signals that mediate the timing of puberty and sexual behavior in male mice. The signals for some, if not all, of these effects in both males and females are detected in the vomeronasal organ. These pheromonal effects were unique in our knowledge of mammalian reproduction when they were discovered, but we now appreciate that there are similar pheromones in many mammals.

In recent years scientists have tried to associate the physiological and behavioral responses in reproduction with specific compounds isolated from mouse urine. We will note some difficulties shortly, but first we

should mention some of the successes. Several studies directed toward isolation of volatile components come from Milos Novotny, an expert in applications of gas chromatography, and his collaborators at Indiana University. Since 1980 scientists have recognized that female urine does not suppress puberty in a young female if the urine comes from females whose adrenal glands have been removed. Presumably, synthesis of the urinary pheromone is under control of hormones produced by the adrenals, and when these hormones are lacking, the pheromone is no longer synthesized. With this in mind, Novotny and his co-workers compared volatile components of the urine of intact and adrenalectomized female mice. Analytical gas chromatography indicated that the levels of certain urinary constituents drop after the adrenals are removed. The chemists were able to isolate and identify six of these constituents. As you can see from their structures, these are relatively simple compounds. When these six compounds are added together at appropriate concentrations to the inactive urine of adrenalectomized females, it exhibits the full activity of normal urine. The mixture of six compounds is also effective when dissolved in water rather than in inactive urine. These six compounds together then act as the pheromone that delays female puberty. A six-

$$CH_3CH_2CH_2CH_2CH_2COCH_3 \qquad CH_3COOCH_2CH_2CH_2CH_2CH_3$$

These structures show constituents of the urinary pheromone of the female house mouse that delays the onset of female puberty.

component signal is complicated in comparison with ones we have seen earlier, but we shall soon meet even greater complexity.

Provoking Aggression

There is also a chemical signal in mouse urine that provokes aggression in male mice, and the team at Indiana carried out a similar search for the compounds responsible for this effect. Male house mice can be trained to fight, and when confronted with a normal male, a trained fighter sniffs, quickly becomes aggressive, and begins to bite and chase the other mouse. Castrated males, on the other hand, arouse little aggression in fighters. If an investigator rubs urine from a normal male onto a castrated male, however, a fighting male will attack just as vigorously as if the other mouse were a normal male. Urine from a castrated male does not have this effect. These observations indicate that the aggression-provoking pheromone is in the urine and that for the animal to synthesize the pheromone, its testes must be intact. (In the wild, house mice live in communities in which one male is dominant. The other males are all subordinate to this dominant male and seem to have no hierarchy among themselves. The dominant male exerts his authority over the others forcefully, and many of them carry bite wounds from frequent encounters with him.)

The urine of normal and castrated males was analyzed by gas chromotography, and it was found that the concentration of two components differed greatly in the two samples. These were 2-*sec*-butyldihydrothiazole and dehydro-*exo*-brevicomin. When these compounds were added in the proper concentrations to castrate urine, the urine became a signal that induced aggression in fighting

males. (Earlier, we met *exo*-brevicomin, the compound with a single bond in place of the double bond of dehydrobrevicomin, as a component of an aggregation pheromone in bark beetles. The skeleton of brevicomin is not a common one, and it seems odd to find these two closely related substances in such diverse species as the house mouse and bark beetles. No one has offered an explanation for this peculiarity.)

Novotny and his group learned more about these compounds and the pheromone that arouses aggression in fighting males. Castrate urine treated with only one of the two compounds remained inactive, and the two compounds together showed no bioassay activity when dissolved in water rather than urine. These and other results suggest that in addition to both identified components, the entire complex odor of castrate urine may be necessary to elicit aggressive behavior. In this case, the two identified components are required but have no activity by themselves.

This is slightly different from the case of the hamster attractant pheromone. In that case one compound, dimethyl disulfide, accounts for much of the attractivity of the vaginal discharge in the bioassay, but only the combination of dimethyl disulfide and all the other volatiles provides full attractivity. Scientists have also found pheromones in which no individual components are absolutely necessary and no components are individually active, but recombination of all the volatiles recreates the pheromone.

2-*sec*-Butyldihydrothiazole   Dehydro-*exo*-brevicomin

We can call olfactory signals arising from large numbers of components complex odors. For the first time we face the possibility that an olfactory signal simply may not be referable to one or a few compounds. This complexity offers a substantial obstacle to chemical studies of mammalian pheromones, and we must turn our attention to this matter before leaving the mammals. This also gives us an opportunity to discuss in more detail a class of extraordinary chemical signals that we have mentioned only briefly up to now. These are recognition pheromones, the signals that identify individuals or sets of individuals.

Complex Odors and the Scents of Individuals and Groups

There are some natural scents, such as those of wintergreen, caraway, or bell peppers, that are reasonably approximated by single chemical compounds. However, there are other very familiar smells that simple mixtures of compounds cannot even crudely imitate. The aromas of chocolate, coffee, tea, and wine come to mind as examples. All of us can easily identify each of these aromas, yet each is subject to infinite variation. Professionals routinely distinguish large numbers of different wines by bouquet. These distinct odors can result from minute differences in chemical composition, and this makes exhaustive analysis difficult.

An analogous situation exists with certain mammalian pheromones, and progress toward complete chemical identification of these signals has been slow. As mammals with their elaborate brains exchange more refined and varied messages, the chemical nature of some of the signals employed grows more complex and less amenable to thorough description.

Many of these complex odors are signals that facilitate individual or group recognition. We have already suggested that in two species each member of a population has a unique scent. The young black-tailed deer recognizes its mother by sniffing and licking her tarsal tufts. Urine from a strange male house mouse prevents implantation and pregnancy in a recently inseminated female. There are many other mammals whose perception of individual or group odors has been proved experimentally or inferred from their behavior. There is good evidence that lemurs (both *Lemur fulvus* and *Lemur catta*) and saddle-back tamarins *(Saguinus fuscicollis)* can recognize individual odors, and there are less rigorous indications of the same thing in old-world monkeys and apes.

Individuals or families of many species mark their territories with a chemical signal, usually in urine or feces, that others of their kind perceive and respect. Individual recognition and its practical consequences have a long history in animal husbandry. Nursing ewes routinely reject all lambs but their own after one or two sniffs, and sheep men must adopt elaborate ruses to induce foster mothers to accept orphan lambs. There is no chemical information yet about these signals. Learning plays an important role here, and the specific odor of an individual or a group is obviously quite different from a pheromone used regularly throughout a species.

While we cannot yet analyze these signals chemically, there has been some inquiry into their origins. One possibility is that an identifying scent is picked up directly from others. For example, after a few days of suckling a foster mother, an orphan lamb acquires a scent, presumably from her milk, that makes it henceforth acceptable to the ewe.

Another possible source of individual or group odors is genetic differences. Each organ-

An adult spotted hyena *Crocuta crocuta* and a dark-furred cub sniffing each other. For many species of mammals sniffing is a common means of identifying individuals and groups.

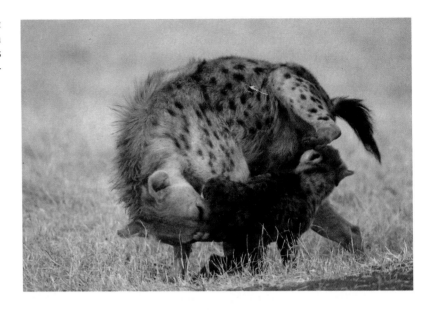

ism carries its own unique biological and chemical blueprint in its genes, and we might suppose that some part of this plan pertains to the signalling of individuality. In fact, Lewis Thomas of Memorial Sloan-Kettering Cancer Center in New York suggested in 1974 that a set of genes found in all vertebrates and known as the major histocompatibility complex (MHC) might be responsible for individual odors. MHC genes direct the synthesis of proteins that are carried on the surface of cells, where they indicate the origin and condition of the cell. From these indicators the immune system can determine whether a cell is part of the organism or a foreigner. Cells that are recognized as healthy and part of the organism itself are ignored. Sick cells and foreign invaders are destroyed. Owing to their association with individual identification, MHC genes have received much attention in studies of tissue transplantation. MHC compatibility between human donor and recipient, for

example, is crucial to the success of kidney transplants. MHC genes also appear to affect matters quite close to our present interests. The efficacy of strange-male pregnancy block in mice has been linked to the MHC types of the particular male and female in question. Moreover, there are statistically significant differences in the volatile constituents of the urine of mice belonging to two different MHC types. These include both major differences in the concentrations of a few components and also more subtle shifts in the ratios of many other components.

These signs of a connection between MHC genes and the recognition of identity aroused the interest of investigators at the Monell Chemical Senses Center in Philadelphia and the Memorial Sloan-Kettering Cancer Center. They performed a very pretty experiment showing that an almost unbelievably minute difference in the MHC genes carried by different individuals can lead to a variation in urinary odor. For this experiment they used two carefully bred populations of mice. All the mice in each group were believed to be genetically identical except for one MHC gene. This gene supplies the code that specifies the sequence of the amino acids in a particular protein. The two versions of the MHC gene carry the code for proteins whose chemical structure is nearly, but not quite, the same in the two populations of mice. The scientists determined the sequence of amino acids in each of the two versions of this protein and discovered that in a series of more than 400 amino acids the two proteins differed in only three amino acids. The very small change in the genetic code for this protein necessary to alter these three amino acids is the only known genetic difference between the two populations of mice.

Now, what interests us here is that, in a bioassay, other mice were able to discriminate between these two nearly identical populations by the odor of their urine. This difference in odor presumably arises from the single genetic difference. Between the slight variation in one protein that this difference introduces and the ultimate effect on the odor of urine, there must be a multitude of biochemical events about which we know nothing. Nonetheless, the experiment argues that a tiny genetic difference can suffice to alter a smell associated with identity. Genetic differences can govern individual scents. Other factors doubtless in-

fluence individual and group scents, and there is no reason to expect a single explanation for these signals. While the lamb may get its characteristic smell from the ewe's milk, the individual odor of the milk could be dictated by the ewe's genes.

Complete chemical decoding of the messages borne by complex odors will probably depend upon new techniques. One promising approach is the application of computerized pattern recognition to analysis of these complex signals. This technique permits comparison of the concentrations of the many components of related signals and identification of possible patterns of composition. As these patterns are not necessarily apparent on simple inspection, this analysis can lead to discovery of subtle similarities and differences in the composition of related signals. More generally, an overall solution to the problems of chemical communication in mammals also demands progress in understanding mammalian behavior and in the neurophysiology of olfactory perception and processing. Certainly, none of this will be trivial.

The challenges offered by mammalian pheromones are attractive to many investigators, perhaps because with mammals they find themselves close to home. Perhaps, too, behind an enthusiasm for mammalian pheromones there lies a fundamental curiosity about pheromones in humans. In our final chapter we take a look at this topic.

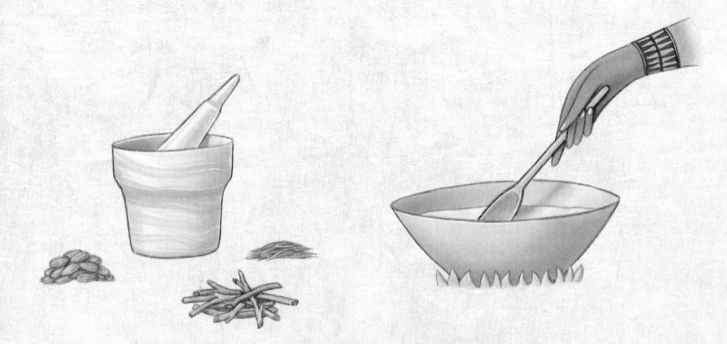

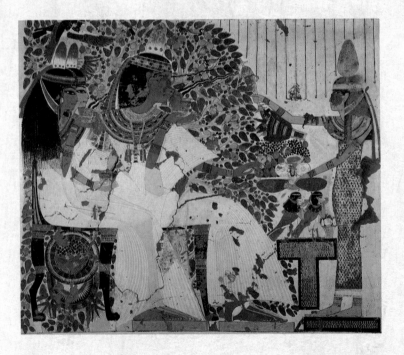

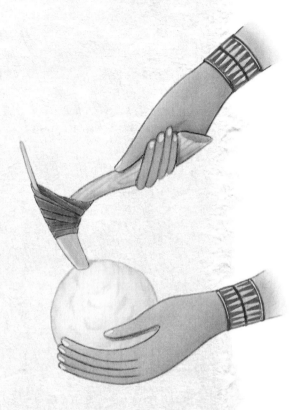

7

HUMAN
ATTRACTIONS

■ An Egyptian wall painting depicts a family entertained in a garden, wearing on their heads cones of animal fat scented with fragrant plant resins. During the warm evening, each cone would melt and trickle down the guest's face and neck. These cones were manufactured by grinding herbs, cooking the herbs with animal fat and resins, then shaping the cooled, solid unguent with an adze. Our ancient fascination with perfumes suggests an intriguing connection between perfumes and pheromones in humans.

*W*e arrive at last at a question that intrigues us all. What about pheromones in humans? From what we have already said about human beings and other mammals, you can probably anticipate part of the answer. All of the problems introduced by the mammalian brain and complex odors are still with us, and to these we now must add those complicating characteristics of human life such as pervasive intelligence, culture, individual and group experience, and language. The very attributes that make us human pose serious obstacles for identifying the effects of chemical signals. Furthermore, for humans olfaction is greatly overshadowed by vision and hearing. We are a long way from the typical nocturnal mammal that finds the world a rich source of chemical signals. The very fact that we pose the question about human pheromones reflects an uncertainty concerning their importance for us. From what has gone before and from our own experience, we expect pheromones to be less significant for humans than for deer or hamsters, and we anticipate that, if pheromones exist in our species, there may be real obstacles to obtaining experimental data about them. We can now be more explicit.

If the question about pheromones in humans means, "Is there a behavioral imperative in humans comparable to that of the hamster mounting pheromone?" the answer has to be that it seems most unlikely. Even among nonprimate mammals, hamsters are peculiar in depending completely on olfaction to stimulate

normal sexual behavior. Human sexual behavior is notoriously complex in both basis and expression, and there is no reason to assume that someone is going to isolate an aphrodisiac chemical signal bearing an urgent and irresistible message for humans. This is not to say that the possibility of less compelling aphrodisiacs can be rigorously dismissed.

There is no hard evidence, but a positive view of this matter comes from a report famous in the nineteenth-century psychosexual literature and repeated many times since. This concerns a young Austrian peasant who carried his handkerchief in his armpit and used it with thoughtful solicitude to wipe the faces of his local dancing partners. By all accounts, his amorous adventures met with enviable success unapproached by his peers. After our discussions later of perfumes and axillary odors, you may decide that the young Austrian took unfair advantage of his lady friends. Perhaps so,

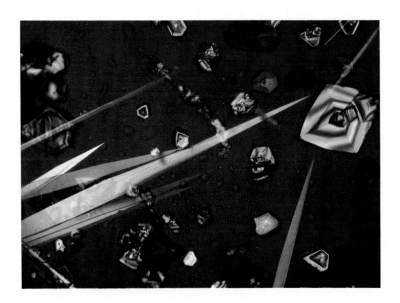

The major human sex hormones as they appear in crystalline form under a polarizing microscope. The male's hormone testosterone forms sharp needle-like crystals, while the female's estrogen makes small clumps called rhomboids.

but it is doubtful that his handkerchief carried a chemical signal that deserves all the blame. I suspect that he was also an exceedingly persuasive young man.

If the question about pheromones in humans means, on the other hand, "Is there chemical communication of any sort in humans?" the answer is more affirmative. We will discuss information about several sorts of signals that reflect the present state of evidence for human chemical communication.

Prostaglandins as Possible Pheromones

Prostaglandins turned up earlier in our story as a hatching pheromone in the arctic barnacle and as the postovulatory pheromone of the goldfish. We noted that both invertebrates and vertebrates possess this group of compounds, which serve a wide range of physiological functions. Prostaglandins of several kinds are found in humans, and in fact this whole family of substances was first discovered in the 1930s in human semen. Their synthesis in the seminal vesicles of men is regulated by testosterone, but their precise role in semen is not yet established.

Prostaglandins stimulate contractions of the human uterus, and this may be one of their important functions in seminal fluid. These uterine contractions may help sperm move to the fallopian tube where fertilization takes place. If prostaglandin-induced contractions do facilitate human reproduction in this way, prostaglandins qualify as pheromones. This is a situation that we have not encountered before: we are certain about the occurrence, biochemistry, and chemistry of prostaglandins, and we know they cause uterine contractions in humans. What we do not

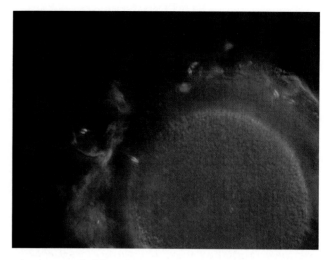

This remarkable photomicrograph has captured a human sperm just as its head penetrates the egg. Has a pheromone emitted by the egg guided the sperm to its goal?

yet know is whether these contractions perform a significant function, qualifying prostaglandins as pheromones, or are merely incidental.

A Possible Sperm Attractant

In early 1991 a collaborative team of scientists in Israel and the United States reported suggestive evidence for an attractant that guides human sperm to the egg for fertilization. Only a few hundred sperm cells out of perhaps three hundred million that start the trip finally move up the fallopian tube to the site of fertilization. These final competitors may be swimming up a concentration gradient of pheromone released by the egg or nearby cells. From women undergoing in vitro fertilization, the investigators obtained samples of the fluid that surrounds the fertilizable egg. They observed that many more sperm swam to this fluid than to a control solution. This strongly suggests that a chemical signal is attracting the sperm. If the scientists can prove this suggestion and isolate the responsible pheromone, this discovery could be important in the treatment of infertility and in new approaches to contraception.

In early 1992 support for this idea of a sperm attractant came from Dr. Marc Parmentier at the Free University of Brussels and his colleagues. These investigators discovered about twenty different olfactory receptors in sperm tissue. The receptors were the same kind of protein molecules that detect odors in the nose, and they were not found in several other types of tissue, such as kidney and liver. No one knows yet what these sperm olfactory receptors do or why there are so many different kinds of them, but they may receive chemical signals that guide the sperm on its long journey to the egg.

Mother-Infant Recognition

Charles Darwin recorded more than a century ago that an infant with its eyes closed will turn its head toward its mother's breast when it is brought near. He suggested that the infant was responding either to the mother's odor or to her body heat. Experiments in recent years have demonstrated that during the first six weeks of life infants show an increasing preference for the smell of their mother's breast over that of another mother. Most likely the infant has learned to recognize the scent of its mother during these first weeks after birth. This scent may include not only the mother's innate odor but also the infant's own odor, which has been transferred to the mother during suckling. In this way the infant may effectively mark its mother for future recognition.

There is evidence that the reverse process, the ability of a mother to identify her infant, becomes established more rapidly. One group of investigators examined mothers and infants immediately after delivery. They blindfolded each mother and presented her with her own child and two other newborn babies. In 61

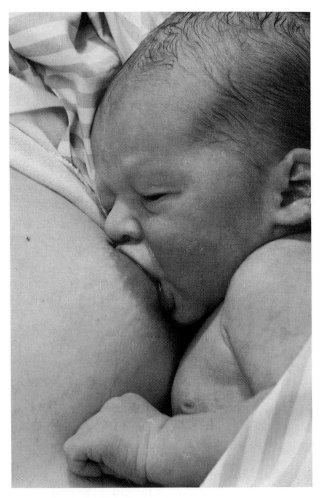

A breast-feeding infant becomes familiar with its mother's odor and also transfers its own odor to her.

percent of the trials the mother correctly identified her own baby, much better than the 33 percent expected by chance. In a similar experiment fathers attempting to recognize their own children within two days of birth were correct only 37 percent of the time, little better than the result of random choice. Other investigators have shown that children can recognize their siblings, and parents can recognize their children, by the smell of clothes they have worn. Also, both men and women can discriminate their own body odor from that of others. As in other mammals, all these feats of identification presumably rely upon odors that are highly individual and quite complex. These recognition phenomena are well-documented instances of chemical communication in humans.

Menstrual Synchrony

Groups of women living together often exhibit menstrual synchrony. College women residing in the same dormitory and also family units of mother, daughters, and sisters have encountered and commented on this experience for many years. Typically on coming together a body of women have menstrual cycles randomly scattered throughout the month, but after several months of communal living their cycles coincide within a period of a few days. This phenomenon is reminiscent of the discovery that pheromones from a group of female mice influence estrus in another female.

Menstrual synchrony in women was first investigated by Martha K. McClintock at Harvard University (now at the University of Chicago). She followed the menstrual cycles of 135 college undergraduates living in a dormitory at a suburban women's college. During the period from October to April menstrual

synchrony gradually imposed itself among groups of close friends and roommates, but not throughout the population of the dormitory. McClintock examined several possible causes for her findings, including the subjects' common diet, their habitual eating together, similar life patterns and shared periods of stress, possible common exposure to periods of light and dark, and their awareness of the timing of one another's cycles.

Her data permitted rejection of all of these potential explanations. Moreover, there was no relationship of age or college year to the patterns of synchrony that emerged. The single identified factor that did correlate with synchrony was the amount of time the subjects spent together. The women who spent the most time with one another tended to come into menstrual synchrony. A second finding in this study, also reminiscent of prior observations in the mouse, was that those women who spent time with men most often (three or more times a week) had shorter and more regular menstrual cycles. McClintock announced these results in 1971, and they stimulated considerable interest in the prospects that pheromones could regulate menstruation in humans.

In 1986 experimental evidence for this hypothesis appeared. George Preti and his collaborators at the Monell Chemical Senses Center and the University of Pennsylvania reported a careful study suggesting that female axillary (underarm) sweat is the source of a chemical signal leading to menstrual synchrony. A group of women who had regular menstrual cycles served as "donors." These women kept careful records of their menstrual cycles and collected their axillary sweat on pads three times a week through three complete menstrual cycles. Preti then pooled the pads in batches, so that each batch consisted of pads from a three-day portion of the donors' cycles. One batch was for days one, two, and three, another for days four, five, and six, and so forth, to make a total of ten batches. (All the donors had cycles of 29 ± 2 days.) Preti and his colleagues then applied these batches of axillary sweat sequentially to a separate set of women we will call the recipients. They prepared an alcoholic solution from each batch of pads and applied a small amount of one of these solutions to the upper lip of each recipient three times a week. Each recipient received axillary odors progressively through the menstrual cycle of the donors. A control group received only applications of alcohol as a stimulus. After 10 to 13 weeks of this treatment the menstrual cycles of the recipients had shifted significantly toward the timing represented by the test stimuli. No shift had taken place in the cycles of the controls. Something in the axillary sweat of the donors changed over their menstrual cycles and altered the timing of the recipients' cycles.

The investigators at the Monell Center carried out a parallel study using male axillary sweat. They collected sweat from men and prepared an extract in alcohol just as before. They then applied this male extract in a similar fashion to a set of women selected for their long or short cycles (fewer than 26 or more than 32 days). After 12 to 14 weeks of regular exposure to the male extract, the cycles of these women had approached the normal cycle length of 29.5 ± 3 days. No such effect occurred in controls that received only alcohol. Something in male axillary sweat acts as a chemical signal to govern the regularity of menstruation.

Both male and female axillary sweat have demonstrable pheromonal effects on menstruation, and this provides an explanation for McClintock's observations. We do not yet know what chemical compounds are responsible, but these two investigations by Preti and his colleagues are probably as firm evidence as we now have for pheromones in humans.

Why did these investigators choose to examine axillary sweat as a potential source of chemical signals? The underarm area differs structurally from surrounding portions of the human body in two relevant ways. The skin here contains tiny secretory structures called apocrine glands, and in most races it also supports a relatively extensive growth of hair. The apocrine glands become active at puberty and then begin to contribute their secretion to axillary sweat. The association of apocrine glands with abundant hair is widespread in mammals, and for many species these glands serve as major sources of chemical signals. The tarsal gland on the hind leg of the black-tailed deer, for example, contains many apocrine glands and has a conspicuous tuft of hair. We have seen that this structure is the source of a variety of socially significant pheromones. The hair increases the surface area coated with the apocrine secretion that is exposed to the atmosphere; hence the secretion's volatile components are dispersed more efficiently into the surroundings. Scientists had suggested that apocrine glands might be a source of chemical signals in humans as well. With a knowledge of the importance of apocrine secretions, it was natural for Preti and his co-workers to concentrate their attention on axillary sweat.

Perfumes, Musky Odors, and Pheromones

Preti's discovery of chemical signals in axillary sweat connected human odors experimentally with reproductive physiology. However, humans had apparently made this connection much earlier in a nonscientific way, as we shall see on examining the ancient use of perfumes and incense. This examination will also hint at a surprising connection between perfumes and human pheromones.

For thousands of years perfumery has linked fragrance with sex, or more broadly, with human emotion. The Assyrians and Egyptians burned vast quantities of incense in their religious and political ceremonies. The Greeks and Romans did the same, both on public occasions and in their private homes. In biblical times spices scented both the marriage bed and the funeral bier. (We have a catalogue of the aromatic substances that Moses carried on leaving Egypt, and many of these are still in general use.) Characters in Shakespeare rubbed civet on their bodies as a perfume. In context, all these activities heighten an occasion or improve the status of an individual.

Whatever the original reasons for the use of perfumes, our interest in them has been thoughtfully nurtured and encouraged over the years. Playing on human anxieties and the universal desire to enhance our individual power and attractiveness before an often indifferent world, purveyors of perfume through the ages have urged upon us the considerable advantages of smelling good. Modern advertisements

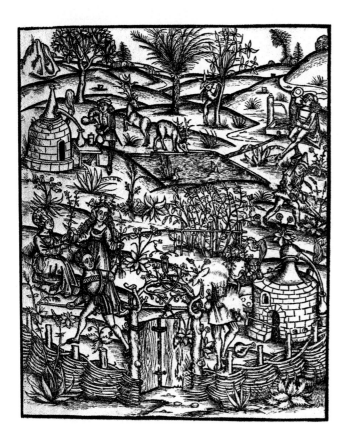

"Herb Garden and Distillery," from Hieronymous Brunschweig's *Liber de arte Distillandi de Simplicibus* (1516). The aromatic waters could be distilled from herbs such as lavender, elderflower, and rosemary and used as perfumes, or herbs could be ingredients in more complex perfumes. One of Queen Elizabeth's favorite perfumes was made of rose water and damask water boiled with powdered sugar, to which was added dried sweet marjoram and powder of gumresin benzoin. The recipe yielded a dry powder, which was carried in little bags kept in the pocket.

A male musk deer. Adult males have a gland in their abdomen that secretes a brownish waxlike substance prized since antiquity as a source of musk. For centuries the species has been vigorously hunted for the small amount of secretion yielded by each deer. Although musk remains in great demand, the musk deer has been saved from extinction probably by its retiring habits and the discovery of alternative sources of musk.

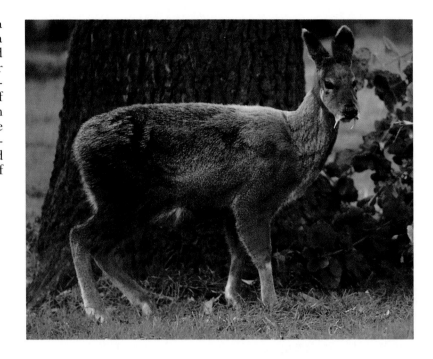

for perfumes make delicious promises, in pictures if not in words. The right fragrance will overcome inevitable personal shortcomings in intelligence, beauty, wealth, or whatever, and we can come out on top smelling like a rose. Whether or not we find this argument compelling and delight in dabbing ourselves with perfume or after-shave lotion, it seems obvious that perfume has met some elementary need of varied races and cultures across millennia of human history.

Two of the oldest-known ingredients of perfumes, musk and civet, are odoriferous animal products that function as attractant pheromones in nature. Musk originally came from the male musk deer *Moschus moschiferus*, a native of China and Tibet, while the sources of civet were the African and Asian civet cats *Viverra civetta* and *Viverra zibetha*. Both musk

and civet were ancient articles of commerce. The Koran speaks of a paradise populated with "black-eyed houris [nymphs] . . . of the purest musk." These fragrances were exotic imports to Europe from the East, and, in fact, the words *musk* and *civet* both came into European languages from the Persian names for the substances.

Musk and civet have a heavy, musky odor that is still considered essential in perfumery. Through the years cheaper and more convenient natural sources of musky scents were found. Not only more accessible mammals, such as the muskrat, provided appropriate substitutes, but there were also an octopus, an alligator, and a snail that furnished musky essences; there is even a musk beetle. Twentieth-century chemical investigations of the active principles of musk and civet and the subse-

quent laboratory preparation of these compounds permitted synthetic chemicals to
replace the animal products. The major active
compounds in natural musk and civet are two
large-ring compounds known as muscone and
civetone. Most of the rings in natural products
contain five or six carbon atoms, and these
compounds with fifteen- and seventeen-
membered rings are distinctly odd.

The musky note of other types of natural
aromas is also valued in perfumery. One such
article of commerce is sandalwood oil, which
comes from an Indian evergreen
(Santalum album). This oil has a pleasant,
sweet-woody odor with a shade of a musky or
urinous overtone. The two main components
are α- and β-santalol, compounds that are
structurally unrelated to muscone and
civetone.

Why should perfumery prize mammalian
chemical signals that smell musky? We lack a
detailed history of the early human use of
musk and civet, but the outlines of a fascinat-

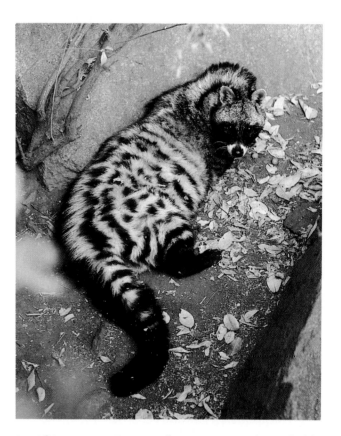

An African civet. Despite their savage and unreliable
disposition, African civets were traditionally kept in
large stockades in East Africa and regularly "milked."
The strong-smelling secretion of a complex scent
gland near the anus was removed, packed into cow
horns, and sold at a high price to perfumers around
the world.

Muscone

Civetone

ing speculation are visible in what we have already said. This explanation finds an underlying relationship between these musky compounds and a group of odoriferous steroids. You may recall the steroids that give boars their musky breath and function as a pheromone to induce lordosis in the sow. These and related steroids are also minor components of human sweat that are produced by bacteria from steroids secreted by the axillary apocrine glands. Both male and female sweat contain these steroids, although their concentration is considerably higher in males. As we know, pheromones in this sweat influence the timing of the human menstrual cycle.

It is very tempting to propose that the musky steroids are active components of these human pheromones. After all, these compounds are both present in the sweat and already proved pheromones in other mammals. If musky steroids are human pheromones, then perhaps other musky compounds also have some pheromonal effect in humans. Perhaps there is even a specific olfactory receptor for compounds that we perceive as musky, so that other musky smells can mimic the pheromonal effect of the natural signals. The messages of these pheromones could have influenced our forebears more openly than they do us, but maybe such compounds still account for the age-old human interest in musk and civet. You can see that it all sounds perfectly possible and makes a beguiling tale. In fact, there are experimental investigations that support some aspects of this line of thought, but at present the overall idea remains an engaging speculation.

Related ideas could also explain the historical origins of perfume and incense. Where did this fashion for modifying the smell of people and their surroundings come from? Nowadays, perfumes ostensibly replace or mask our natural body odor, which our cul-ture deems embarrassing and offensive. Perhaps originally perfumes did not mask, but rather *enhanced*, our human smell. In a more primitive and less fastidious world, maybe humans desired the pheromonal advantages of their natural body odors. Perhaps they discovered that they could fortify their own musky pheromone with substances borrowed from other creatures and learned to value natural musks for this property. While conscious memory has rejected this initial purpose of perfumes, the fundamental reasoning could still be correct and account at a deeper level for the status of perfumes even today. This entire concept was nicely summarized half a century ago in the psychoanalytic literature with the proposition that perfumes "unconsciously reveal what consciously they aim to hide." The notion is too intriguing to dismiss, but for now it too remains a speculation.

Problems for the Future

We began with a look at chemical signals disseminated by simple organisms, such as water molds and brown algae, and moved from there through the animal kingdom, finding chemical signals all along the way. High points appeared in the insects and the mammals, where the social organization of many species demands extensive communication between individuals. It is probably also true that scientists have conducted a more widespread search for pheromones in these two classes than elsewhere. Chemical communication is an indispensable aspect of the existence of many diverse creatures.

With apparently millions of extant species not yet even described, future chemists and biologists can no doubt continue to search out and study specific pheromones for as long as they wish. Methods and techniques are in

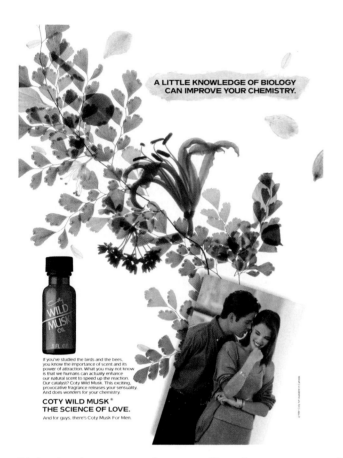

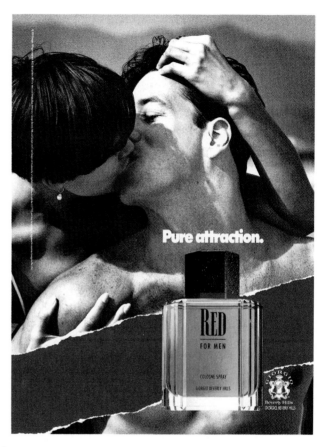

Right: A cologne spray for men offers the enticement of "pure attraction." *Left:* "Wild Musk Oil" for women. According to the advertisement, "If you've studied the birds and the bees, you know the importance of scent and its power of attraction. What you may not know is that we humans can actually enhance our natural scent to speed up the reaction. . . . This exciting and provocative fragrance releases your sensuality. And does wonders for your chemistry."

place, and we know in general terms how to identify both the compounds that act as pheromones and the responses that they elicit. Beyond this level, however, there are major problems not yet solved. We have already spoken of complex odors in this regard.

There are also more fundamental experi-

mental limitations to extending our understanding of pheromones, and two present constraints can serve as examples. Pheromones will turn up in unexpected places as we refine methods for the isolation, purification, and identification of smaller and smaller amounts of chemical compounds. The steroids in human sweat were identified in picogram amounts, which is roughly the current limit for identifying such compounds. What would we learn if we could routinely isolate and identify compounds in femtogram or attogram amounts? (One femtogram is one one-thousandth of a picogram or 1×10^{-15} gram; one attogram is one one-millionth of a picogram or 1×10^{-18} gram.)

On the biological side, we are hampered by our limited comprehension of olfaction. How do organisms discriminate odors? Olfaction in mammals is particularly difficult to study, owing to complicating factors that we have discussed. We still know very little about how the brain handles olfactory signals, and the human brain remains one of the great problems for scientific investigation. Our current state of biological knowledge of nearly all pheromones is that a signal goes into the olfactory or accessory olfactory system, and a behavioral or physiological response comes

out. What would we learn if we could examine all the steps in the nervous system between the arrival of pheromones and the responses to their messages?

Today we simply do not know the answers to these questions, but we are moving toward their solution. An exciting biological advance came in April 1991, when Linda Buck and Richard Axel of Columbia University, working with rats, identified a large family of genes that appear to control the synthesis of olfactory receptor proteins. One immediate implication of this finding is that the number of these receptor proteins is surprisingly large. The discovery will permit biologists to begin working out details of the structure and function of the receptor proteins. With this information we will begin to understand chemically how olfaction works. The next few years could bring dramatic advances in this area. Our understanding grows broader and deeper all the time.

GLOSSARY

alcohol An organic compound containing a hydroxyl (—OH) group.

algae A large group of chiefly aquatic, nonvascular organisms containing chlorophyll. Examples are seaweeds and pond scums.

amino acid As used here, one of the twenty common naturally occurring small molecules that are strung together to form peptides and proteins. All have a nitrogen atom adjacent to a carboxyl group:

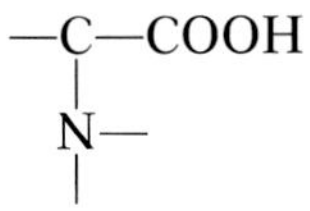

$$
\begin{array}{c}
\text{—C—COOH} \\
| \\
\text{N—} \\
|
\end{array}
$$

attogram 1×10^{-18} gram. For more information see **units of measurement.**

axilla The armpit.

bioassay A procedure for estimating the amount of a biologically active preparation, such as a pheromone, in a sample by monitoring the sample's biological effect on an organism. When fractionation techniques are used to purify a pheromone, the bioassay identifies the fraction containing the active substance. For more detail, see page 9.

carbohydrate A chemical compound formed from one or more sugars joined together.

carbonyl group The functional group

$$
\begin{array}{c}
\text{O} \\
\| \\
\text{—C—}
\end{array}
$$

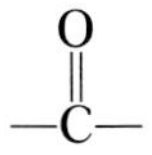

composed of a carbon atom doubly bonded to an oxygen atom; frequently written —CO—.

carboxyl group The functional group

$$
\begin{array}{c}
\text{O} \\
\| \\
\text{—C—OH}
\end{array}
$$

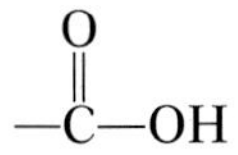

composed of a carbonyl group bonded to a hydroxyl group; frequently written —COOH.

compound A substance made up of units, each of which contains a specific combination of atoms. Molecular compounds consist of molecules; ionic compounds consist of ions with an equal number of positive and negative charges.

concentration gradient As used here, the roughly regular change in concentration of a chemical compound or mixture with change in distance from its source.

cuticle An outer covering layer of many organisms, typically hard or tough.

diploid Having a double set of chromosomes, which is the common condition of body cells.

double bond A functional group that consists of two atoms joined by two bonds. When both atoms are carbon, these two atoms and the four attached groups all lie in a single plane. Owing to the rigid planar nature of the double bond, there are two possible arrangements of the attached groups, creating two different substances, a Z form (from the German *zusammen*, together) and an E form (from the German *entgegen*, opposed). Older names for these two forms are *cis* and *trans*, respectively.

Z form   E form
(cis)   (trans)

drone A male bee.

enzyme A protein that facilitates a biological reaction without itself being altered or consumed.

ester A compound that contains the functional group

$$-\overset{\overset{\text{O}}{\|}}{\text{C}}-\text{OR}$$

where R is a hydrocarbon group; often written —COOR.

estrus A regularly recurrent state of sexual excitability during which the female will accept the male and is capable of conceiving. The related adjective is *estrous*.

fatty acid A compound made up of a hydrocarbon chain terminating in a carboxyl group. Some fatty acids contain double bonds.

femtogram 1×10^{-15} gram. For more information see **units of measurement.**

fractionation The systematic separation of a mixture of chemical compounds into its pure components. This is done by taking advantage of differences in the chemical and physical properties of these components. In working with

pheromones, a bioassay normally guides progress in this activity. For more detail, see page 9.

functional group A group of two or more atoms bonded together that brings characteristic physical and chemical properties to a compound.

fungi A large group of nonvascular organisms that absorb food from other organisms and do not contain chlorophyll. Examples are mushrooms and yeasts.

gas chromatography A technique for separating volatile compounds on the basis of solubility and volatility.

gamete A reproductive cell. Male gametes are sperm cells; female gametes are egg cells.

gonad A gland that produces gametes. In animals the male gonads are the testes, which produce sperm, and the female gonads are the ovaries, which produce eggs.

hormone A chemical compound produced in an organism and transported to another part of the organism, where it produces a behavioral or physiological effect.

hydrocarbon A compound or a functional group containing only carbon and hydrogen atoms.

hydroxyl group The functional group —OH.

hyphae The interconnected threads that make up the body of certain water molds and fungi.

intromit Insert, specifically to insert the penis into the vagina.

ion An atom or group of atoms that carries an electrical charge.

Lepidoptera The group of scaly-winged insects, including butterflies and moths.

lipids A class of compounds including fats, oils, and waxes that consist largely of esters formed by uniting fatty acids that have long chains with alcohols or other molecules.

mass spectrometry A physical technique that furnishes information on the size and chemical structure of molecules, usually through breaking the molecules apart by bombardment with electrons. See also the illustration on page 21.

methyl The group

$$\begin{array}{c} \mathrm{H} \\ | \\ -\mathrm{C-H} \\ | \\ \mathrm{H} \end{array}$$

It is often written $-\mathrm{CH_3}$.

microgram 1×10^{-6} gram. For more information see **units of measurement.**

milligram 1×10^{-3} gram. For more information see **units of measurement.**

molecule A discrete grouping of atoms in a specific three-dimensional arrangement.

nanogram 1×10^{-9} gram. For more information see **units of measurement.**

odorant A volatile chemical compound responsible for an odor.

organic As used in chemistry, this term means containing carbon. Organic compounds contain carbon atoms, and organic chemistry is the chemistry of these compounds.

ostariophysians The group of about 5,000 bony fishes that includes the great majority of the freshwater species. Typical members are minnows, carps, and catfishes.

ovary The gland that produces female gametes.

ovulation The discharge of eggs from an ovary.

peptide A molecule made by joining two or more amino acids together. A peptide of specific length may be called a dipeptide (two amino acids), tripeptide (three amino acids), etc. A peptide with many amino acids is a polypeptide. Above about thirty or forty amino acids, such a molecule is called a protein. A typical dipeptide is

$$\mathrm{CH_3-CH-\overset{\overset{\displaystyle O}{\|}}{C}-NH-CH_2-\overset{\overset{\displaystyle O}{\|}}{C}-OH}$$
$$\underset{\mathrm{NH_2}}{|}$$

picogram 1×10^{-12} gram. For more information see **units of measurement.**

protein A chemical compound composed of many amino acids joined together. Proteins may contain hundreds or even thousands of amino acids.

receptor A protein molecule with which a pheromone, hormone, or other molecule interacts in delivering a message.

sessile Permanently fixed, immobile.

solubility The amount of a compound that will dissolve in a given quantity of another compound or mixture of compounds. Like other physical properties of chemical compounds, solubility is determined by structure.

solvent A liquid compound or mixture of compounds in which other substances are dissolved.

spawn To deposit eggs; applied to aquatic animals.

spectroscopic techniques Various measurements of physical properties, particularly the absorption of light, of chemical compounds or mixtures of compounds that provide information about structure and purity. From these measurements, investigators can frequently determine the complete chemical structure of a compound.

structural formula A two-dimensional representation of the three-dimensional structure of a chemical compound.

structure The specific three-dimensional arrangement of atoms joined to form a molecule. The structure is what differs from one compound to another; specifically, what differs are the number and kind of atoms involved, the order in which these atoms are joined, their arrangement in space, and the type of bond joining each pair of bonded atoms. The structure is responsible for the unique chemical and physical properties of each chemical compound.

synthesis The process of building up a specific molecule from simpler molecules through chemical transformations. Chemists perform syntheses in the laboratory, and organisms perform syntheses in their cells.

taxonomic classification Biologists organize organisms into groups having similar characteristics. Every species of organism, both living and extinct, belongs to a genus (plural *genera*), family, order, class, phylum (or division), and kingdom, with extra levels of classification frequently employed for further clarification (subclasses and superorders, for example). Many similar families belong to the same order, and many similar orders belong to the same class. For most of the organisms discussed in the text the genus and species are given. Usually just enough more of its complete classification is included to give an idea of the relative location of the organism in the living world. It is customary to italicize the name of both genus and species and to capitalize the name of the genus but not the species. For example, the systematic name of the temperate-zone honey bee is *Apis mellifera*. It is the species *mellifera* in the genus *Apis*. This genus also includes several other species of honey bee. It and related genera belong to the Apidae, the bee family, which is in the order Hymenoptera. This order embraces bees, wasps, and ants. The Hymenoptera are one of the orders making up the class Insecta, which includes all the insects. The class Insecta belongs to the phylum Arthropoda, which also includes crustaceans, arachnids, and several other classes. The phylum Arthropoda is in the kingdom Animalia, along with all other animals.

testis (plural, *testes*) The gland that produces male gametes.

units of measurement Scientists use the metric system to express mass and length. The basic unit for mass is the gram (28.35 grams is 1 ounce), and the basic unit for length is the meter (1 meter is 39.37 inches). For convenience a system of standard prefixes is attached to these units to indicate multiples or fractions of the basic measure. The prefixes of interest here, along with their meanings, are milli- (1×10^{-3}), micro- (1×10^{-6}), nano- (1×10^{-9}), pico- (1×10^{-12}), femto- (1×10^{-15}), and atto- (1×10^{-18}). Thus, a milligram is one one-thousandth of a gram, and a micrometer is one one-millionth of a meter. Ordinary grains of salt or sugar have a diameter of roughly 0.2 to 0.5 millimeter or 200 to 500 micrometers. Grains of salt weigh roughly 0.1 to 0.5 milligram or 100 to 500 micrograms.

volatile Able to vaporize at a relatively low temperature.

water molds Funguslike microorganisms that are widespread in freshwater environments.

zygote The cell formed by the union of sperm and egg.

FURTHER READING

Most of these articles are reviews or general discussions that contain numerous references to original papers. Some articles assume a more extensive background in animal behavior, biology, or chemistry than I have assumed in the text.

General Reading and Chapter 1

General

Burton, R. *The Language of Smell*. Boston: Routledge and Kegan Paul, 1976.

McGraw-Hill Encyclopedia of Science and Technology. New York: McGraw-Hill, 1987.

Norris, D. M., ed. *Perception of Behavioral Chemicals*. Amsterdam: Elsevier, 1981.

Prestwich, G. D., and G. J. Blomquist. *Pheromone Biochemistry*. Orlando, Fla.: Academic Press, 1987.

Bacterial response to chemicals

Koshland, D. E., Jr. *Bacterial Chemotaxis as a Model Behavioral System*. New York: Raven Press, 1980.

Anosmia

Ackerman, Diane. *A Natural History of the Senses*. New York: Random House, 1990.

Amoore, J. E. "Olfactory Genetics and Anosmia." In *Chemical Senses: Olfaction*, edited by L. M. Beidler. Berlin: Springer Verlag, 1971.

Pheromones in plants

Baldwin, I. T., and J. C. Schultz. "Rapid Changes in Tree Leaf Chemistry Induced by Damage: Evidence for Communication Between Plants." *Science* 221 (1983): 277.

Rhoades, D. F. "Responses of Alder and Willow to Attack by Tent Caterpillars and Webworms: Evidence for Pheromonal Sensitivity of Willows." In *Plant Resistance to Insects*, edited by P. Hedin. Washington, D.C.: American Chemical Society, 1982.

Chapter 2

Pheromones in *Allomyces*

Pommerville, J. "The Role of Sexual Pheromones in *Allomyces*." In *Sexual Interactions in Eukaryotic Microbes*, edited by D. H. O'Day and P. A. Horgan. New York: Academic Press, 1981.

Pheromones in *Achlya*

McMorris, T. C. "Antheridiol and the Oogoniols, Steroid Hormones Which Control Sexual Reproduction in *Achlya*." *Phil. Trans. Roy. Soc. Lond.* B 284 (1978): 459.

Riehl, R. M., and D. O. Toft. "A Sex Steroid Receptor in the Water Mold *Achlya ambisexualis*. In *The Receptor*, edited by P. M. Conn. Orlando, Fla.: Academic Press, 1986.

Pheromones in brown algae

Müller, D. G. "The Role of Pheromones in Sexual Reproduction of Brown Algae." In *Algae as Experimental Systems*, edited by A. W. Coleman et al. New York: Alan R. Liss, 1989.

Pheromones in *Streptococcus faecalis*

Clewell, D. B., et al. "Sex Pheromones and Plasma-related Conjugation Phenomena in *Streptococcus faecalis*." In *Streptococcal Genetics*, edited by J. J. Ferretti and R. Curtiss III. Washington, D.C.: American Society for Microbiology, 1987.

Chapter 3

Sperm attractants in invertebrates

Miller, R. L. "Sperm Chemo-orientation in the Metazoa." In *Biology of Fertilization*, edited by C. B. Metz and A. Monroy. Orlando, Fla.: Academic Press, 1985.

Pheromones in nematodes

Huettel, R. N. "Chemical Communicators in Nematodes." *J. Nematol.* 18 (1986): 3.

Pheromones in the blue crab

Gleeson, R. P. "Intrinsic Factors Mediating Pheromone Communication in the Blue Crab, *Callinectes sapidus*." In *Crustacean Sexual Biology*, edited by T. Bauer and J. W. Martin. New York: Columbia University Press, 1991.

Pheromones in ticks and mites

Sonenshine, D. E. "Pheromones and Other Semiochemicals of the Acari." *Ann. Rev. Entomol.* 30 (1985): 1.

Pheromones in scorpions

Polis, G. A., ed. *The Biology of Scorpions*. Stanford, Calif.: Stanford University Press, 1990.

Pheromones in spiders

Pollard, S. D., A. M. Macnab, and R. R. Jackson. "Communication with Chemicals: Pheromones and Spiders." In *Ecophysiology of Spiders*, edited by W. Nentwig. Berlin: Springer Verlag, 1987.
Stewart, D. M. "Endocrinology of Arachnids." In *Endocrinology of Selected Invertebrate Types*, edited by H. Laufer and R. G. H. Downer. New York: Alan R. Liss, 1988.

Chapter 4

General

Bell, W. J., and R. T. Cardé, eds. *Chemical Ecology of Insects*. Sunderland, Mass.: Sinauer Associates, 1984.
Blum, M. S. "Biosynthesis of Arthropod Exocrine Compounds." *Ann. Rev. Entomol.* 32 (1987): 381.
Payne, T. L., M. C. Birch, and C. E. J. Kennedy, eds. *Mechanisms of Insect Olfaction*. Oxford: Clarendon Press, 1986.
Peters, T. M. *Insects and Human Society*. New York: Van Nostrand Reinhold, 1988.

History of the identification of bombykol

Hecker, E., and A. Butenandt. "Bombykol Revisited—Reflections on a Pioneering Period and on Some of Its Consequences." In *Techniques in Pheromone Research*, edited by H. E. Hummel and T. A. Miller. New York: Springer Verlag, 1984.

From pheromone to behavior in a moth

Hildebrand, J. G. "From Semiochemical to Behavior: Olfaction in the Sphinx Moth, *Manduca sexta*." In *Molecular Entomology*, edited by J. H. Law. New York: Alan R. Liss, 1987.

Alkaloid-derived pheromones

Eisner, T., and J. Meinwald. "Alkaloid-derived Pheromones and Sexual Selection in Lepidoptera." In *Pheromone Biochemistry*, edited by G. D. Prestwich and G. J. Blomquist. Orlando, Fla.: Academic Press, 1987.

Pheromones in bark beetles

Birch, M. C. "Aggregation in Bark Beetles." In *Chemical Ecology of Insects*, edited by W. J. Bell and R. T. Cardé. Sunderland, Mass.: Sinauer Associates, 1984.

Use of pheromones in pest control

Ridgway, R. L., R. M. Silverstein, and M. N. Inscoe, eds. *Behavior-modifying Chemicals for Insect Management*. New York: Marcel Dekker, 1990.

Orchid mimicry of bee and wasp sex attractants

Van der Pijl, L. and C. H. Dodson. "Mimicry and Deception." Chapter 11 in *Orchid Flowers: Their Pollination and Evolution*. Coral Gables, Fla.: University of Miami Press, 1966.

Pheromones in bees

Free, J. B. *Pheromones of Social Bees*. London: Chapman and Hall, 1987.
Wheeler, J. W., and G. C. Eickwort. "Semiochemicals of Bees." In *Chemical Ecology of Insects*, edited by W. J. Bell and R. T. Cardé. Sunderland, Mass.: Sinauer Associates, 1984.

Pheromones in ants

Hölldobler, B., and E. O. Wilson. *The Ants*. Cambridge, Mass.: The Belknap Press of Harvard University Press, 1990.

Howse, P. E. "Semiochemicals of Ants." In *Chemical Ecology of Insects*, edited by W. J. Bell and R. T. Cardé. Sunderland, Mass.: Sinauer Associates, 1984.

Chapter 5

General

Duvall, D., D. Müller-Schwarze, and R. M. Silverstein, eds. *Chemical Signals in Vertebrates*. New York: Plenum Press, 1986.
Macdonald, D. W., D. Müller-Schwarze, and S. E. Natynczuk, eds. *Chemical Signals in Vertebrates 5*. New York: Oxford University Press, 1990.

Pheromones in the blind goby

Bardach, J. E., and J. H. Todd. "Chemical Communication in Fish." In *Communication by Chemical Signals*, edited by J. W. Johnston, D. G. Moulton, and A. Turk. New York: Appleton-Century-Crofts, 1970.

Courtship in salamanders

Houck, L. D. "The Evolution of Salamander Courtship Pheromones." In *Chemical Signals in Vertebrates*, edited by D. Duvall, D. Müller-Schwarze, and R. M. Silverstein. New York: Plenum Press, 1986.

The vomeronasal organ

Cooper, W. E., and G. M. Burghardt. "Letter to the Editor." *J. Chem. Ecol.* 16 (1990): 103.
Duvall, D. "A New Question of Pheromones: Aspects of Possible Chemical Signaling and Reception in the Mammal-like Reptiles." In *The Ecology and Biology of Mammal-like Reptiles*, edited by N. Hotton et al. Washington, D.C.: Smithsonian Institution Press, 1986.
Meredith, M. "Trigeminal Response to Odors." In *Sensory Systems: Senses Other than Vision*, edited by J. M. Wolfe. Boston: Birkhäuser Boston, 1987.

Pheromones in the red-sided garter snake

Crews, D., and W. R. Garstka. "The Ecological Physiology of a Garter Snake." In *Scientific American*, 247 (November 1982): 159–168.

Garstka, W. R., and D. Crews. "Pheromones and Reproduction in Garter Snakes." In *Chemical Signals in Vertebrates*, edited by D. Duvall, D. Müller-Schwarze, and R. M. Silverstein. New York: Plenum Press, 1986.

Mason, R. T., and D. Crews. "Pheromone Mimicry in Garter Snakes." In *Chemical Signals in Vertebrates*, edited by D. Duvall, D. Müller-Schwarze, and R. M. Silverstein. New York: Plenum Press, 1986.

Pheromones in birds

Wenzel, B. M. "The Ecological and Evolutionary Challanges of Procellariiform Olfaction." In *Chemical Signals in Vertebrates*, edited by D. Duvall, D. Müller-Schwarze, and R. M. Silverstein. New York: Plenum Press, 1986.

Chapter 6

General

Albone, E. S. *Mammalian Semiochemistry*. Chichester: John Wiley, 1984.

Brown, R. E., and D. W. Macdonald, eds. *Social Odours in Mammals*. Oxford: Clarendon Press, 1985.

Duvall, D., D. Müller-Schwarze, and R. M. Silverstein, eds. *Chemical Signals in Vertebrates*. New York: Plenum Press, 1986.

Novotny, M. "The Importance of Chemical Messengers in Mammalian Reproduction." In *Masculinity/Femininity: Basic Perspectives*, edited by J. M. Reinisch, L. A. Rosenblum, and S. A. Sanders. New York: Oxford University Press, 1987.

Stoddart, D. M. *The Ecology of Vertebrate Olfaction*. New York: Chapman and Hall, 1980.

Vandenbergh, J. G. "Pheromones and Mammalian Reproduction." In *The Physiology of Reproduction*, edited by E. Knobil and J. D. Neill. New York: Raven Press, 1988.

Individual odor in primates

Epple, G., A. Belcher, K. L. Greenfield, I. Kuederling, K. Nordstrom, and A. B. Smith III. "Scent Mixtures Used as Social Signals in Two Primate Species." In *Perception of Complex Smells and Tastes*, edited by D. G. Laing et al. Orlando, Fla.: Academic Press, 1989.

Salivary pheromone of the pig

Gower, D. B., and W. D. Booth. "Salivary Pheromones in the Pig and Human in Relation to Sexual Status and Age." In *Ontogeny of Olfaction*, edited by W. Breipohl. Berlin: Springer-Verlag, 1986.

Chapter 7

General

Ellis, H. *Studies in the Psychology of Sex*, Vol. 2, 44. New York: Random House, 1936.

Stoddart, D. M. *The Scented Ape*. Cambridge: Cambridge University Press, 1990.

Prostaglandins

Moore, P. K. *Prostanoids: Pharmacological, Physiological, and Clinical Relevance*. Cambridge: Cambridge University Press, 1985.

Perfumery

Leach, M., ed. *Standard Dictionary of Folklore, Mythology, and Legends*. New York: Funk and Wagnalls, 1950.

Theimer, E. T., ed. *Fragrance Chemistry*. New York: Academic Press, 1982.

Van Toller, S., and G. H. Dodd, eds. *Perfumery*. London: Chapman and Hall, 1988.

SOURCES OF ILLUSTRATIONS

Illustrations rendered by William C. Ober and Claire Garrison of Medical and Scientific Illustration and Fineline Illustrations, Inc.

Page 28
D. G. Müller. From I. Maier and D. G. Müller,
"Sexual Pheromones in Algae," Biol. Bull. *Vol.*
170, page 145, 1986.

Page 29
left, J. Robert Waaland/Biological Photo Service
right, D. G. Müller. From I. Maier and D. G. Mül-
ler, "Sexual Pheromones in Algae," Biol. Bull. *Vol.*
170, page 145, 1986.

Page 30
Reinhard Wirth

Page 32
George Lepp/Comstock

Page 35
D. Wrobel MBA/Biological Photo Service

Page 36
Lovell and Libby Langstroth

Page 37
Norbert Wu

Page 38
Jack Clark/Comstock

Page 39
R. N. Huettel and R. W. Reise, USDA/ARS, Belts-
ville, Maryland

Page 42
Norbert Wu

Page 46
E. A. Janes/NHPA

Page 47
Richard B. Forward, Duke University

Page 50
Lilia Ibay de Guzman, Dept. of Entomology, Loui-
siana State University, Baton Rouge and the
USDA/ARS Honey-Bee Breeding Genetics and
Physiology Laboratory

Page 53
Runk/Schoenberger/Grant Heilman Photography

Page 53
Adapted from G. S. Habicht, Gregory Beck, and
Jorge L. Benach, "Lyme Disease," Scientific American, *Vol. 257, (1), pages 78–83, July 1987.* © *1987*
by Scientific American, Inc. All rights reserved.

Page 56
John Shaw

Page 58
Edward Ross

Page 61
Peter Bryant/Biological Photo Service

Page 62
left part of figure from Figure 8.13 in David
Freifelder, Physical Biochemistry, *W. H. Freeman*
and Company, 1976.

Page 63
R. A. Steinbrecht

Page 64
Photograph by Erich Hecker. From E. Hecker and
Adolf Butenandt, "Bombykol Revisited—Reflections
on a Pioneering Period and on Some of Its Conse-
quences." A. Butenandt et al., Techniques in Pheromone Research, *New York, Springer, 1984.*

Page 66
From W. L. Roelofs, CHEMTECH, *Vol. 9, page*
222, 1979.

Page 70
left, Peter Byrant/Biological Photo Service

Page 68
Adapted from Dietrich Schneider, "The Sex Attract-
ant Receptor in Moths," Scientific American, *Vol.*
231, (1), pages 28–35, July 1974. © *1974 by Scien-*
tific American, Inc. All rights reserved.

Page 70
right, Thomas Eisner

Page 71
Maria Eisner, Cornell University

Page 72
Adapted from Figure 2.4a and b, page 25, in Forest Insects: Principles and Practice of Population Management *by Alan A. Berryman, Plenum Press, New York, 1986.*

Page 73
Jack Clark/Comstock

Page 74
Jack Clark/Comstock

Page 75
right half of figure from Figure 4, in Lloyd E. Browne, Martin C. Birch, and David L. Wood, Journal of Insect Physiology *(1974) Vol. 20, page 188, Pergamon Press PLC, 1974.*

Page 79
David Maitland/Planet Earth Pictures

Page 80
Trécé Incorporated, Salinas, California

Page 82
Jack Clark/Comstock

Page 84
from Cassell PLC, Villiers House, London, England

Page 85
Edward Ross

Page 87
Kenneth Lorenzen

Page 90
Kenneth Lorenzen

Page 91
Edward Ross

Page 93
Edward Ross

Page 95
From Figure 14, page 126 in W. Hangartner, Z. Vergleich. Physiol. Vol. 57, page 103, 1967.

Page 96
painting by John Dawson, © National Geographic Society

Page 98
Heather Angel/Biofotos

Page 100
Heather Angel/Biofotos

Page 101
Agence Nature/NHPA

Page 104
left part of figure from K. von Frisch, "Die Bedeutung des Geruchssinnes im Leben der Fische," Naturwiss. *Vol. 29, pages 321–333, 1941.*

Page 106
Heather Angel/Biofotos

Page 112
Philip Chapman/Planet Earth Pictures

Page 115
Brian Milne/First Light

Page 118
Adapted from David Crews and William R. Garstka, "The Ecological Physiology of a Garter Snake," Scientific American, *Vol. 247, (5), pages 163–168, November 1982. © 1982 by Scientific American, Inc. All rights reserved.*

Page 122
Michael Leach/NHPA

Page 124
Frans Lanting/Minden Pictures

Page 125
Anthony Bannister/NHPA

Page 126
Russ Kinne/Comstock

Page 130
Art Wolfe

Page 133
Adapted from R. D. Estes, "The Role of the Vomer-onasal Organ in Mammalian Reproduction," Mammalia, *Vol. 36, pages 315–341, 1972.*

Page 134
Erwin and Peggy Bauer/Wildstock

Page 136
From Figure 1 in A. G. Singer et al., "Dimethyl Disulfide: An Attractant Pheromone in Hamster Vaginal Secretion," Science *Volume 191, page 949, 5 March 1976, ©AAAS.*

Page 142
Stephen Dalton/NHPA

Page 146
Frans Lanting/Minden Pictures

Page 148
Egyptian Expedition of the Metropolitan Museum of Art, New York. Rogers Fund, 1930. (30.4.33).

Page 150
Lennart Nilsson, A Child is Born, *Dell Publishing Co.*

Page 151
Lennart Nilsson, A Child is Born, *Dell Publishing Co.*

Page 152
Lennart Nilsson, A Child is Born, *Dell Publishing Co.*

Page 156
Mandal Ranjit/NHPA

Page 157
J. P. Scott/Planet Earth Pictures

Page 159
left, © Giorgio. Reproduced by permission.
right, Pfizer Inc., Coty Division. Reproduced by permission.

INDEX

Other books in the Scientific American Library Series

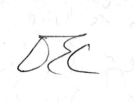